Praise for *Birth:*

"A startling journalistic take on birth practices over the centuries . . . Fascinating."
—*FitPregnancy*

"This history of childbirth is both a literary and a medical history achievement and belongs in any library strong in either medicine or feminist perspectives. An outstanding survey, this moves beyond the usual medical focus into the lives and experiences of woman giving birth."   —*The Midwest Book Review*

"A must for every pregnant woman's bookshelf . . . Brave, inspiring, and occasionally laugh-out-loud funny—a bit like childbirth itself."
—Viv Groskop, *Sunday Express* (London)

"A wonder of a book. The history of birth, as Cassidy deftly tells it, might well be summed up as What No One Ever Expected When They're Expecting. . . . With wit and aplomb, Cassidy covers the ongoing march of birthing fads, from the surreal horrors of the Twilight Sleep to Lamaze, doulas, and the current craze for elective C-sections. A must read for anyone who's ever been born."
—Mary Roach, author of *Stiff: The Curious Lives of Human Cadavers* and *Spook: Science Tackles the Afterlife*

"It's as true of feminism as anything else that if we don't know our history we're condemned to repeat it. A liberating look at how assumptions have changed of what a good childbirth is supposed to be."
—Naomi Wolf, author of *The Beauty Myth* and *Misconceptions*

"A rich cultural history of the subject."   —*The Philadelphia Inquirer*

"As Tina Cassidy describes it in *Birth*—and she is persuasive—our choices about where, how, and even when to give birth are guided, if not limited, by a culture that shapes us much more than we realize. . . .[*Birth*] has real value for women who want to understand why the reality of giving birth didn't match their careful plans and expectations."   —Alexandra Bowie, *The New York Sun*

"Well-written and will be an important eye-opener to many."— *Publishers Weekly*

"Tina Cassidy's *Birth* is a fascinating ride through centuries of childbirth practices—from the days when midwives reigned to the dawn of male doctors, from the modern natural-birth movement to the astronomical increase in C-sections—and all the bizarre gadgets and lore in between. Cassidy's spirited writing makes this historical account read like a compelling novel."   —Melissa Chianta, *Mothering*

"Replete with interesting facts about the physiology, politics, and pieties of birth across the ages."   —*Daily Press*

Birth

The Surprising History
of How We Are Born

Tina Cassidy

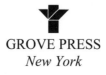

GROVE PRESS
New York

Published simultaneously in Canada

Printed in the United States of America

Library of Congress Cataloging-in-Publication Data

Cassidy, Tina.

   Birth : the surprising history of how we are born / Tina Cassidy.

   p. cm.

   Includes bibliographical references (p. 285)

   ISBN-10: 0-8021-4324-5

   ISBN-13: 978-0-8021-4324-2

   1. Childbirth—History. I. Title.

   RG651.C37 2006

   618.2—dc22   20006047589

Grove Press
an imprint of Grove/Atlantic, Inc.
841 Broadway
New York, NY 10003

Distributed by Publishers Group West

www.groveatlantic.com

08 09 10 11 12   10 9 8 7 6 5 4 3

For the Damaschi women and the Flint boys

CONTENTS

IN THE BEGINNING

AFTER I HAD a baby in 2004, the women of my family gave me three things: newborn outfits, advice, and accounts of their own birth experiences.

The last was the impetus for this book.

My grandmother, Genevieve Damaschi, who bore three girls in the 1940s and '50s, explained how she was gassed during the birth of her first daughter, slipping in and out of consciousness on a stretcher in the hallway of Hartford Hospital. She screamed. The nurses told her to "shut up." She didn't see the baby for three days, per standard hospital infection-prevention policy. My grandfather was barred from the room while she labored.

My mother, who had me in 1969, recounted in a ten-second sound bite an equally frightening story of her five-hour labor and delivery ordeal.

"They shaved my pubic area. They gave me an enema. They made me walk around the room a couple of times. They gave me a shot. I woke up three hours later standing on the gurney in excruciating pain. The doctor came in, gave me another shot, and then the next thing I know, you were born."

"Did they use forceps?" I asked.

"I think that they did, because of the condition that your head was in."

"You don't *know* if they used forceps?"

"I'd like to get those records," she said, sounding sort of dreamy, her mind stuck in the labor room where she, too, delivered alone, no husband or family allowed. "Scopolamine," she said. "It makes you not remember what happened. I pretty much slept through it."

When she was about to have my brother in 1976, my mother skeptically attended Lamaze classes, which then were in vogue. There she learned how to breathe—hee hee huhhhh—and her husband was prepped to witness the birth, a relatively new idea at the time. Though her "natural" delivery of me should have been proof that she could deliver this second child vaginally, her doctor gave her an X-ray to determine if her petite pelvis could allow for my brother to pass through. The doctor said her pelvic width was borderline and after just a couple of hours of normal labor, suggested a cesarean section. Unhappy with her first birth experience, she leaped at the opportunity. Spouses were almost never allowed in the operating room then. So my mother delivered alone. Again.

My youngest aunt had her first child in 1982, just as natural childbirth methods were peaking, a feminist backlash against the highly controlled births my mother and grandmother had gone through. Hers was the most unusual of all the Damaschi women's labors to date, because her husband witnessed the whole event. But the birth of her second child, in a Catholic hospital in 1989, did not go as well as the first. Because of long-held religious beliefs that it is a woman's station in life to suffer during labor—says so right there in the Bible—the facility did not allow for any pain relief. She was left alone in a room for hours, the baby facing backward in the birth canal, and she tore mightily at the end.

Despite all, I had high hopes for how the birth of my son, at a major hospital in the medical mecca of Boston, would unfold. I purposely chose a female obstetrician. Armed with a birth plan, the latest fad in obstetrical empowerment, I knew I would sail through labor wearing my favorite black spaghetti-strap night-gown—no johnnie for me! The lights would be dim, an epidural anesthetic juicing my spine only if absolutely necessary. I had written down my instructions for the nurses to read so that even if I was in too much pain to explain it to them myself, my plan would be clear.

An instructor at the hospital's prenatal class told us that the episiotomy, a cut to make the opening of the birth canal wider, was no longer routinely performed by their obstetricians because they now knew that the incisions often caused more problems than they solved. The doctors also had abandoned stirrups because they had learned that having women lie flat with their legs in the air negates the powerful force of gravity for pushing out the baby. They said they didn't routinely employ forceps anymore, which can in-jure the mother and child. And the doctors had stopped objecting to squatting, which opens the pelvis, an ancient practice that had been rediscovered after disappearing in the prudish Victorian era.

My husband and I felt blessed to have the latest thinking at our disposal. But after ten hours of labor and another four hours of pushing, the very busy obstetrician making rounds that night told us matter-of-factly that our son had not rotated all the way, and was stuck. I asked to have a midwife come and offer sugges-tions to move my labor along, but the harried staff said she was unavailable. I asked them to shut off the epidural (yes, I had suc-cumbed the fifth time the nurse asked me if I wanted one), so that I could try other labor positions. They obliged but only, I think, because they were annoyed and knew the pain would be so severe I wouldn't care what happened next. Indeed, that was true.

My son's heart rate was fine, but things had dragged on too long, as far as the staff was concerned. The doctor insisted upon an emergency C-section—which was performed with the speed of a SWAT team—throughout which I vomited and shook vio-lently, while my poor husband clung to my side of the operating

3

curtain, careful not to glimpse my uterus, which rested outside my abdomen while the doctor stitched it. The next morning, my still-ashen spouse, grateful everyone was alive and the baby was perfect, cornered the doctor, wanting to know if the ordeal had really been necessary.

"What did they do in that situation before there were C-sections?" he wanted to know.

"The baby would have died in the birth canal," the doctor said. "They would have had to wait for it to disintegrate, or they would try to get it out some other way, drilling a hole in the fetal head, emptying the contents and collapsing the skull, before it started to poison the mother."

Well, then.

I caught this response as I shuffled out of the bathroom on my way back to bed. Too weak to react, I gingerly climbed beneath the blanket and filed a mental note to see if that was true. If I had lived five hundred years ago . . . I drifted into a fitful, clammy, bloated sleep, my body pumped even larger with fluids than it had been before the birth, while little George, softer and sweeter than heaven, lay wrapped up like a burrito in the crook of my arm, where I longed to keep him forever.

I was in a great deal of abdominal pain; it hurt more than I could endure to get in and out of bed. The doctor, following standard procedure, had cut through my taut belly skin, through a layer of fat, cauterizing along the way, until she reached the fascia, the glistening sheet, which looks like the filmy layer on a chicken breast, that undergirds the abdominal wall. She then nicked the fascia with the knife and extended the cut with scissors, pushing, not cutting, to tear the tissue like a sheet of wrapping paper. Once the fascia was peeled away, she pulled apart the muscles in the middle, poked a hole with her finger through a layer of tissue underneath, and stretched it hard. Using a clean knife, she cut ever so gently, and not too deep, into my uterus. She pulled apart the incision until it was big enough for the baby's head and reached in elbow deep for the baby's chin as an assistant pushed down hard from the top of the uterus. Someone, I'm not sure who, went between my legs and up inside my body to give him an extra boost before George popped out explosively, rather like a champagne cork.

I may have been in the hospital for the obligatory four long days, but there was no time to be a patient. I was a mom completely in love with my son, awed by him and stunned by how he came into the world, but I was also the primary food source for this amazing little organism, whose needs were constant and exhausting. I was discharged for home feeling utterly drained, my hormones roiling, my body viciously assaulted. All the while a nasty germ was breeding in the incision, forcing a trip back to the hospital, where an obstetrician prodded me with a Q-tip—incredibly, inside the wound—before sending me home in tears with an antibiotic prescription. Next came mastitis, a breast infection typical among novice nursing women.

So much for birth and nursing being "natural" processes. Surely, nature did not intend for any of this to be so difficult. If it did, how could the human race have survived? Was I being a spoiled, wimpy modern woman? Was that why so many of my friends were having similar experiences? And if so, why are some women delighted by the whole affair, from first contraction to final push? Was my son too big? Was I too small? Were my boobs too sensitive? Should I not have succumbed to an epidural?

I've been a journalist for half of my life. I've covered Super Bowls and fashion shows, presidential campaigns and inaugurations, mob trials, bank failures, housing bubbles, kidnappings, and terrorism. I tried to make sense of all of those crazy stories by doing research and asking questions, whether it was pressing John McCain on his agenda while riding the Straight Talk Express or interviewing Tom Ford on a rose petal–strewn Milan runway. Through the frigid, blurry January weeks after George was born, I found myself suddenly housebound with time to ruminate—though not with time to cook or take a shower. When George was peaceful, my mind returned to that nagging question: Why is birth such a crapshoot after all this time? I realized that I needed to use my professional skills to understand women's bodies, the process of labor and birth, and the shockingly intense postpartum weeks. I needed to put into perspective my own experience. I needed to know what other women, in other cultures, in other times, had done.

When, finally, my infections had cleared and my scar had hardened into a thick red keloid, I embarked on a mission that became this book.

It began simply enough. Holding babe in arms, I awkwardly started to search the Internet. When I found little to satisfy my curiosity, I dragged myself to the library.

At first I was disappointed to discover that the most recent comprehensive world history of birth had been written more than fifty years ago. Even that, *Eternal Eve,* a British classic by Harvey Graham, was hard to find and badly outdated. There were a couple of more recent books that focused specifically on American child-birth history, and I found plenty of anti-cesarean, pro–breast-feeding polemics, feminist and academic histories of midwives, and surveys of male-dominated obstetrics, but I knew these didn't tell the whole story.

Indeed, much of what lined the shelves were how-to birth and breast-feeding guides, which were even more annoying now than they had been the first time I read them. There was no single source for the information I wanted, and clearly I was not the only one seeking it. The chatter on baby blogs was anxious. Women everywhere wanted answers to the same questions, from what other cultures use for pain relief, to why so many Dutch women give birth safely at home, to whether all women one day will have cesareans.

Continuing my quest, I descended into vaultlike library basements, where the rare book departments and the microfilm rooms always seem to be located. It was in one of these window-less places that I found proof that my doctor wasn't inventing that horrific tale of demise she told my husband: As early as the sev-enth century, desperate people were using hooks to perform cra-niotomies to extract a stuck child.

Suddenly even more motivated, I paged through the brittle parchment of sixteenth-century midwifery books, as well as vintage obstetric texts and hundreds of old periodicals. Eventually, I visited hospitals and birth centers; inspected antique obstetrical instru-ments in museums; attended a HypnoBirthing class; interviewed mothers, fathers, doctors, midwives, childbirth educators, hospital administrators, lawyers, academics, public health activists, and an-thropologists. I spent days with nurses and anesthesiologists, wit-nessed single and multiple births, natural and cesarean. And sought out the latest trends. All to try to understand what is supposed to be a natural—perhaps the most natural—physiological process.

The more I learned, the more questions I had: How did midwives go from being burned as witches to vaunted by yuppies? Who let men in the room? Why would someone give birth in the ocean? What does the *Titanic* have to do with an ultrasound scan? Is there a link between Pitocin and autism? What did Queen Victoria have to do with epidurals? How is a woman's pelvis undermined by eating Big Macs? Were cesarean sections really named after Julius Caesar? Could it possibly be true that even in early twentieth-century America, women delivering in hospitals were more likely to die there than if they had given birth at home? That poor women were used as obstetrical guinea pigs? That doctors use drugs to confine deliveries to banker's hours? That some women have orgasms with vaginal births? (Yes!)

The answers—the surprising, frustrating, tantalizing an-swers—helped me realize that my childbearing experience, like my family's chain of births, was merely a reflection of its time and place. My son's birth may have been just as painful as the drawn-out, agonizing vaginal birth that my mother had for me. At least I was conscious and accompanied.

It is astonishing to me that we can touch the moon and predict the weather, map the human genetic code and clone animals, digitize a photograph and send it from Tokyo to Tehran with the touch of a button, but we can't figure out how to give birth in a way that is—simultaneously and consistently—safe, minimally painful, joyful, and close to nature's design.

As you will see, if history is our guide, we never will figure out the ultimate way to give birth. And we probably will never stop trying. For no matter that birth is the most natural of events, the arrival of a healthy baby is truly a miracle.

1 EVOLUTION AND THE FEMALE BODY

I SPOTTED LUCY, framed and hanging on the walls, in the bowels of the American Museum of Natural History. The three-million-year-old fossilized australopithecine was a creature in mid-evolution between ape and *Homo sapiens*. She is one of the oldest human ancestors ever discovered.

Having just seen the expansive pelvises of knuckle-scraping apes and chimps in other displays in the museum, I was shocked to see Lucy's pelvis, so tiny and elliptical from hip to hip that it could not have been easy for her to give birth, not even if the baby's head was the size of a lemon. Staring at Lucy's remains, I imagined the agony and ecstasy of birth since the beginning of time. And I thought about the connections between her bones and the advent of midwives, epidurals, surgical instruments, medical malpractice claims, a newborn with a cone head, and virtually every trendy technique that has come and gone throughout the centuries. It was clear that if we had ape-sized pelvises, we'd need no midwifery help, no sterilized stainless-steel paraphernalia, and no Demerol to give birth. But there would be other consequences.

Lucy, unearthed in Ethiopia in 1974, was related to those apes and chimps; she had long arms, short legs, and a face with ape-like features. But she was clearly different in one respect. She walked upright. And there was her compact pelvis to prove it. As an evolutionary entry point, Lucy can help explain not just the

9

physical aspects of human birth, which have become remarkably more difficult since we began walking upright and producing smarter offspring with the requisite larger crania, but also how primitive behaviors that may have existed in her era are still affecting labor and delivery today. Since Lucy's lifetime, the female pelvis has remained narrow, so as to accommodate our walking upright, but it also has evolved in shape to accommodate the newborn head, which has grown in size over hundreds of thousands of years as the brain enlarged. Today, the upper opening of the pelvis is wide from side to side, as was Lucy's; the lower pelvis, however, the baby's exit, is widest from front to back. And therein lies the problem.

The obstetrical consequence of such a design is that human birth is, quite literally, a twisted process. In order to pass through the birth canal, the baby's head—the largest part of its body—must rotate as it descends in a grinding pirouette. A baby monkey, on the other hand, does not need to turn: It emerges faceup, having had plenty of room to simply drop down the chute.

The contrast between human births and those of four-legged mammals is stunning. Women have a much more difficult time than, say, polar bears, or the free-ranging howler monkey—which can deliver in about two minutes—as each has plenty of space in her birth canal. In fact, we are the only mammal species that needs assistance to give birth.

Although most animals seek solitude for birth, almost all women in labor ask for help or surround themselves with company. It's as if somewhere, deep inside our brains, we cannot fathom how that baby's big head can make a graceful exit. It's a notion that causes fear, which triggers a cry for help in labor and delivery. According to American anthropologist Wenda Trevathan, such an impulse to call for aid could be an adaptive response to reduce mortality in a species more prone to obstetrical problems. This behavior probably developed around two million years ago, she says, along with the advent of consciousness. Once our brains were advanced enough to know that birth could be dangerous, the onset of labor made us scared. Fear often leads to the release of the hormone epinephrine, also known as adrenaline, which can stop contractions. To alleviate that fear—to keep labor progressing—women began asking for help from people they felt comfortable with: other women. Monkeys in labor often stop contracting when they know a human is watching them. Women aren't necessarily different. After laboring at home for hours, many find their labor stalls when they arrive at the hospital, surrounded by the unfamiliar. The phenomenon is so common that doctors and nurses self-referentially call it "white-coat syndrome." For women, being among strangers can retard labor.

Around the world, solitary human births are virtually unheard of. The exceptions are those peoples whose cultures support and value the concept. For example, women of the Igbo tribe of Nigeria may have a first birth supervised but a later one alone. Female members of the nomadic Pitjandjara tribe of Australia might deliver by themselves, behind the group, if there is no worry of trouble. So, too, do women of the !Kung San hunter-gatherers living in the Kalahari Desert in northeastern Namibia give birth on their own—for it is a sign of strength, esteemed in that culture. The story of a !Kung woman named Nisa is remarkable because it shows how even an uncomplicated birth among a people who encourage solitary delivery can be traumatic.

In the chilly depths of night, early in the twentieth century, Nisa gave birth to her first child in the bush without any help. When Nisa's contractions had begun, she left her husband's village, carrying only a blanket and an animal skin for warmth, walked a short distance, sat down on the sandy earth, and waited.

> I leaned against the tree and began to feel the labor. The
> pains came over and over, again and again. It felt as

though the baby was trying to jump right out. The pains stopped. I said, "Why doesn't it hurry up and come out? Why doesn't it come out so I can rest? What does it want inside me that it just stays in there? Won't God help me to have it come out quickly?" As I said that, the baby started to be born. I thought, "I won't cry out. I'll just sit here. Look, it's already being born and I'll be fine." But it really hurt! I cried out, but only to myself. I thought, "Oh, I almost cried out in my in-laws' village." Then I thought, "Has my child already been born?" Because I wasn't really sure; I thought I might have only been sick. That's why I hadn't told anyone when I left the village. After she was born, I sat there; I didn't know what to do. I had no sense. She lay there, moving her arms about, trying to suck on her fingers. . . . The cold started to grab me. I covered her with my duiker skin that had been covering my stomach and pulled the larger kaross over myself. Soon the afterbirth came out and I buried it.

Somewhat stunned, Nisa left the baby, still attached to the placenta by the umbilical cord, and ran back to the village. When her husband saw her bloody legs, he shouted for his grandmother to go and help cut the cord. The old woman promptly did just that.

According to Marjorie Shostak, a researcher to whom Nisa recounted her story, an uncomplicated delivery reflects a !Kung woman's full acceptance of childbearing: "She sits quietly, she does not scream or cry out for help, and she stays in control throughout the labor. A difficult delivery, by contrast, is believed to be evidence of her ambivalence about the birth, and may even be seen as a rejection of the child."

Thankfully, being alone during delivery is a rarity for most women today.

OVERNIGHT DELIVERIES

Another obstetrical phenomenon that may be an adaptation from primitive times is that mammals commonly labor through the night. The squirrel monkey begins her labor between dusk and dawn. If delivery does not happen before morning, her contractions will stop and begin again after sunset. Natural selection might favor nighttime deliveries for some animals—like the squirrel monkey—that search for food during the day. A female who stops to give birth during such a busy time risks being left behind by her kin. Delivering at night also gives mother and offspring time to recover without the risk of being discovered by predators—or even those in their own social group who might want to inspect the new arrival. (The schedule is flipped for nocturnal animals: They tend to deliver during the day.)

Humans, as well, seem to prefer laboring through the night. But because delivery takes longer for people than for monkeys, women tend to give birth in the morning. Such a pattern may also reflect Lucy's era, when it was advantageous to deliver with fellow tribe members around to provide assistance and protection. Those giving birth in the afternoon would likely have found themselves alone, as the others would have been looking for food. Also, laboring through the quiet of the night may keep the mother relaxed and therefore able to have faster, less complicated births.

But, as you might suspect, behavior that worked well on the savanna two million years ago may not be advantageous now. Most dilating women today arrive at the hospital during the late shift, when the staff is reduced and the least experienced doctors are working. More senior obstetricians have the privilege of working business hours, while exhausted residents, living on pizza and donuts and the occasional nap on a cot, attend to the overnight customers. Some women might be willing to forgive a resident who yawns through her contractions at 3:00 a.m. or rushes to the bed at the last second to catch the baby and cut the cord. However, the dearth of well-rested, experienced doctors working overnight, and the lack of hospital services that are available only during the day, can have devastating consequences.

Babies born late at night have as much as a 16 percent greater chance of dying than babies born between 7:00 a.m. and 7:00 p.m., a 2005 study found. This spike in overnight infant deaths may be attributed to the quality and number of doctors and nurses during those dark hours.

There are other ways that life in the developed world hasn't mixed well with the ancient biological process of birth. Take, for example, modern eating habits. Easy access to food is yielding bigger babies that, no matter how hard they try, simply cannot fit through the standard-issue pelvis. This imbalance is called cephalopelvic disproportion, or CPD in *E.R.* language, and is an increasingly common reason for cesarean sections.

Dietary changes affected obstetrics hundreds of years ago, as well, during the period of rapid industrialization and urbanization, which severed populations from fresh milk, green vegetables, and sunlight. Calcium and vitamin D deficiencies led to a bone disease called rickets, which deformed women's already tight pelvises, resulting in countless deaths for mother and baby. The disease was so pervasive that much of the early research and practice for cesareans involved pregnant women with rickets.

Thinking about all this, I peeled away from the display case of Lucy's bones. The sights and sounds of humanity shuffling across the museum floor suddenly reentered my consciousness. I turned and happily saw the throng of well-fed women inching strollers through the café line. Obviously, children—and their mothers—were today regularly surviving birth. How? These women were all taller than Lucy, who stood less than four feet high; their pelvises certainly were somewhat larger. But their babies' heads are more than twice the size of what they would have been in Lucy's time. Proportionately, we still seemed to be losing the battle with evolution.

Back at home, I phoned Owen Lovejoy, professor of biological anthropology at Kent State University in Ohio and of human anatomy at Northeastern Ohio Universities College of Medicine. Lovejoy often can be found brushing through the dirt at fossil excavation sites around the globe, or sitting on the witness stand in high-profile homicide cases.

"Lucy's pelvis was so small!" I said.

Lovejoy laughed and explained that women today are indeed better off than Lucy was, in purely obstetrical terms, but perhaps not by much.

"Because we have her pelvis, we know something about pelvic evolution among humans," Lovejoy explained. "Lucy's pelvis is beautifully adapted to upright walking, but it's poorly adapted to giving birth to a large-brained fetus. And so between Lucy as a starting point and modern humans, we changed the pelvis—not for bipedality but to get that huge cantaloupe through," he explained.

No wonder birth doesn't always go smoothly. The physical frame leaves little room for error. Lovejoy explained that the birth canal became larger, but, more important, it also became different in shape, with the exit now widest between the pubic bone and the tail bone. As a result, the big head is able to descend through a pelvis fine-tuned for walking, though not easily. Assuming the baby is not breech—being born feet or buttocks first—its head must enter the pelvis facing up toward the pubic bone, with the widest part of its head—ear to ear—lining up with the widest part of the pelvis—hip to hip. But, as mentioned, that has to change quickly. The baby must begin to turn sideways, as much as forty-five to ninety degrees, in order to align its body with the widest pelvic outlet, its head emerging facedown, rather than faceup.

In most cases, babies can navigate the space unaided. But not always. Sometimes the space is just too small and the head is too big, so the aforementioned cephalopelvic disproportion becomes a factor.

Birthing babies with large crania would not be an issue if humans had pelvises like chimpanzees, our closest genetic relatives. But if we had pelvises like chimps, we would also walk like chimps, rocking from side to side as if wearing snowshoes. The stance would be an uncomfortably wide, inefficient, and exhausting means of getting around.

Although women's pelvises are universally narrow compared with those of other primates, they vary enough in shape that there are four categorizations for them. If she is lucky, a woman has a "gynecoid" pelvis, the most common and successful shape for birth because it is the most spacious and round. The other shapes—android, resembling a funnel or a narrow heart similar to a male's pelvis; anthropoid, a thin oval; and platypelloid, with a mildly deformed kidney-shaped brim—can also accommodate a baby, but only if they are simpatico with the child's size.

Brand-new babies may appear tiny, especially in those first days, when their fingernails are perfect little specks and their knees are as sweet and wrinkled as shriveled figs. But it doesn't matter

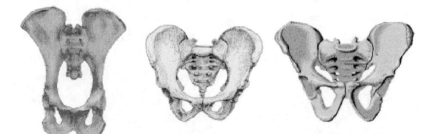

Chimpanzee, Australopithecus africanus, *and* Homo sapiens *pelvises.*

if they're five pounds or eight: Human newborns—and their heads—are proportionately much larger than what other mammals deliver. Female gorillas produce offspring that average only about 2 percent of their mother's weight, compared with 6 percent for humans. Polar bears, who weigh more than five hundred pounds, give birth to cubs with heads smaller than those of human newborns.

Still, anyone who has ever pushed for hours on end only to have the experience culminate in a grapefruit-sized head tearing her flesh might be surprised to learn that while human babies' crania are huge by comparison with those of other animals, their brains aren't as large as they should be.

Lucy's offspring would have needed a tiny head to pass through her small frame. By the later part of the Stone Age, a couple of hundred thousand years ago, the Cro-Magnons appeared in what is now Europe. Their crania—and those of their offspring—had expanded to accommodate all that newfound intellect used to invent religion and draw deer on cave walls using berry juice.

"Brains appear to have gotten bigger progressively throughout the last two million years," said Lovejoy. "But we did hit a wall. The wall we hit was we just couldn't make the pelvis any bigger, so what we had to do is start giving birth to a more altricial infant."

Altricial means that the baby is essentially born helpless. Throughout early human history, brain development made fetal head size grow, but only to the point that it still had a chance to fit through the pelvis. The sorry truth is that babies' crania are actually so small as to be underdeveloped for our species, much more underdeveloped than those of other newborn primates. Human babies compensate by quadrupling brain size after birth. In contrast, most other primate offspring emerge with pretty well-developed brains, having only to double the cranium after birth.

Because human infants are born with their neural networks incomplete, leaving them writhing, helpless squawkers who need constant care during the first year of life, the baby's first three months outside the womb are a period of rapid growth, what many scientists refer to as a fourth "trimester" of development. Other scientists look at infant growth as a two-stage gestation: thirty-eight weeks, followed by thirty-eight weeks outside. Most infants begin to crawl at around nine months of age—the end of the theoretical second stage of gestation—a marker that brings their brains closer to the development level of a deer's when it is born. A deer can run shortly after birth. A baby ape can cling to its mother moments after coming out. But if a human was born with a cranium large enough to make it as developed as the brand-new deer or ape, its head would be too large to fit through the birth canal. For a human baby to emerge as developed as a newborn elephant—which has a 630-day gestation—the child would need to be born with a cranium the size of a one-year-old's, a physical impossibility. Instead, the baby comes out as immature as an infant opossum or kangaroo, which remain protected by a mother's pouch for a long while after birth. It's no wonder tiny babies are cranky. They're really not ready to live outside the womb.

Intelligence and upright walking, the two things that have made human beings so special among mammals, are features that are in direct competition when it comes to survival of the species. Head size may want to expand as we have better nutrition and more doctoral candidates, but nature must keep it in check with pelvis dimensions so we can continue walking on two legs.

"The result of these conflicting requirements," Trevathan writes, "is a species with obstetrical problems and mortality related to birth that is rare among undomesticated animal species."

If we had just *one more inch* of pelvic width, there might be no need for cesareans, forceps, vacuums, and episiotomies. And birthing a baby might not hurt as much. Instead, women and their birth attendants roll the dice virtually every time to see if the parts will align. That leads to a sensible question. Why not eliminate the guessing before labor begins? Can't doctors measure the mother's pelvis and the fetal head well before contractions start or even after they begin? Can't they deduce whether a vaginal delivery will be possible?

TAKING MEASUREMENTS

Scientific attempts to evaluate the width of the birth canal date back to the period of rapid industrialization and urbanization, which severed populations from fresh milk, green vegetables, and sunlight. Calcium and vitamin D deficiencies could lead to the bone softening disease called rickets. At the height of the Industrial Revolution, as much as 60 percent of children living in cold-climate urban areas in Europe and North America had developed the disease, leaving many of them with bowed legs, crooked backs, or warped pelvises, which proved especially dangerous for girls if they ever became pregnant. Two hundred years would pass before researchers determined, in the 1920s, that exposure to sunlight and fortifying the public milk supply with vitamin D helped reduce the incidence of the disease. Rickets is still a problem in less developed countries, especially among darker-skinned peoples and even Muslims, who go about heavily robed. And the problem recently reemerged in the United States, where doctors saw a cluster of rachitic children living in an underprivileged New York neighborhood where they rarely ventured outside out of fear of random violence. Dark-skinned children, in particular, need extra sunlight to help their bodies absorb essential nutrients.

In the eighteenth and nineteenth centuries, doctors used a pelvimeter, an instrument that looked like a giant pair of tweezers with the ends of the pincers curved inward, to determine the size of the birth canal. At the handheld base of the instrument was a measuring device for reading how far the pincers spread out

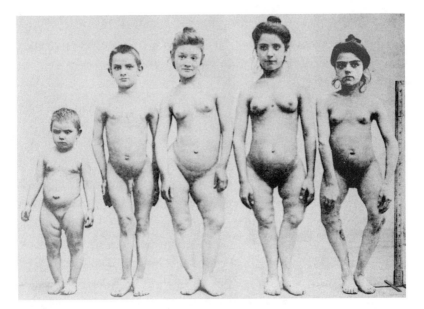

A family with rickets, Paris, circa 1900. (Courtesy the National Library of Medicine)

inside the woman. In some of the worst rachitic cases, the pelvic opening was as small as a quarter.

By the early years of the twentieth century, following German physicist Wilhelm Röntgen's discovery of the X-ray, science had moved on. Doctors soon were using the X-ray not only to measure the fetal and maternal pelvis, but to look for abnormal fetuses, twins, and problems with the placenta, a vital organ created during pregnancy through which the unborn breathes, eats, and filters its waste. Röntgen's technique required the mother to lie on a table while the radiation was zapped in the general direction of the unborn. Though Röntgen won the Nobel Prize in 1901 for his discovery, the medical application was not perfect. The pregnant belly, padded with fat, placenta, and amniotic fluid, put quite a bit of distance between the camera and its subject.

The greater that width, the more distorted the X-ray. Doctors tried to compensate for this by applying an algebraic formula on a simple slide rule. Although X-rays could diagnose extreme situations—twisted pelvises, fetuses with water on the brain—the pictures were not as useful for determining whether an average baby would fit through an average pelvis.

An additional unnerving aspect of this use of X-rays is that doctors were not initially aware that exposure could be harmful to the mother and fetus. When Herman J. Muller first reported in *Scientific Monthly* in 1928 that he was able to mutate fruit flies with x-radiation, doctors began to suspect that the technology could be damaging, especially to developing organisms. By 1942, however, with the advent of new developer processes that required less radiation, X-rays again were proclaimed to be safe. But in 1960, a standard textbook, *Antenatal and Postnatal Care,* sounded the alarm again, saying, "It is now known that the unrestricted use of X-rays may be harmful to mother and child." Two years later, an article in the *Journal of the National Cancer Institute* linked obstetric X-rays to leukemia.

Despite these warnings, X-rays were a tool doctors had come to rely on. And they had nothing with which to replace it—until the now ubiquitous ultrasound came along in the late 1960s. Pregnant women today don't fear that their ultrasounds will cause any harm. Instead, they look forward to the scan with anticipation, learning whether the fetus should be named Louis or Lilah—sometimes there is a Louis *and* a Lilah—and whether there are any abnormalities. The ultrasound can also help narrow a due date and determine whether the late-term fetus is in an awkward position for birth.

As useful as ultrasounds are, they can't predict with a normal pregnancy whether the baby will fit through the exit. For one thing, pregnancy hormones can change the size of the birth canal by loosening ligaments that bind the bones. In rare cases, everything can get so loose down there that the cartilage attaching the two halves of the pelvis at the pubic bone becomes unhinged. Because of these hormones and individuals' differing abilities to stretch, doctors can't predict how much the pelvis will open during labor.

Another unknown is the malleability of the baby's head. The fetal skull has six fontanels, which are soft, membranous areas between the unjoined sections of bony plates. At term, the plates are thin and pliable and often overlap as the head is compressed during the journey through the birth canal. It's impossible to know how much the head will mold—every baby is different.

Despite these uncertainties, modern technology has eased childbirth for millions of women. If only our modern diets could be said to be doing the same.

THE FAST-FOOD PHENOMENON

Whereas Lucy had a diet of nuts, berries, and the occasional piece of meat, her modern descendants are gorging on cheeseburgers, onion rings, ice cream, chips, and whipped cream–topped mocha lattes. There's a fatty, salty, fried, or frozen vice for every maternal desire. And moms aren't the only ones gaining excessive weight during pregnancy. Babies are getting bigger, much bigger, in countries where food and good pregnancy care are plentiful.

According to *Guinness World Records*, Carmelina Fedele of Italy gave birth to the heaviest baby on record. Her toddler-sized infant, born presumably by cesarean in Aversa in 1955, weighed in at 22 pounds, 8 ounces. Of course, the baby was an anomaly, most likely the result of runaway gestational diabetes. But babies in developed countries are indeed being born heavier. Even a cursory check of English-language newspaper stories from 2005 shows how increasingly common jumbo newborns have become, from a Texan named Angel Gabriel (13 pounds, 9 ounces, by cesarean) to English baby Charlie Stokes (15 pounds, 2 ounces, via a "horrific" vaginal birth, according to his mum).

In Australia, a 2002 report found that there had been a 12 percent increase since 1993 in the proportion of babies weighing more than 9.9 pounds at birth. In Ireland, researchers at Dublin's famous Rotunda maternity hospital looked at birth weights for first-time mothers between 1950 and 2000 and found that millennium newborns weighed an average of 7 pounds, 10 ounces, about a pound more than they did a half century earlier. The news is the same across the United Kingdom. A headline in the *Sunday Times* (London) in 2003 announced, "Better British diet gives birth to mega baby." The story said the proportion of babies weighing 9 pounds, 15 ounces, or more, a classification benchmark for large children at birth, rose 20 percent in ten years. A doctor quoted in the piece blamed the drive-through menu, in part, for many of the larger babies.

"Mums with a diabetic tendency and obese mums tend to be more likely to have bigger babies because there is more fat laid down and more sugar present," said Dr. Alan Cameron, a consultant obstetrician at the Queen Mother's hospital in Glasgow. "The fast-food diet also predisposes to increased gestational diabetes, which develops in pregnancy."

In Britain and America, a typical newborn weighs in at about 7 pounds, 8 ounces. Swiss newborns weigh an average of about 8 pounds, with mothers there producing more and more 13 pounders. These are robust infants, compared with those in less developed countries across Asia and Africa. Indian babies, for example, average about 6 pounds.

Why such a boost in birth weight in so short a time? These large babies are not the result of evolutionary changes, which could take thousands of generations to permanently alter human physiology; rather, they are by-products of the rapidly shifting environmental and cultural landscape. Between 1920 and 1975 three generations of women dieted throughout their pregnancies to make sure they did not gain more than the 15 to 20 pounds their obstetricians advised, knowing larger babies came with a big price. It wasn't until the late 1970s that doctors relaxed weight gain limits, acknowledging that if a pregnant woman was hungry, her fetus probably needed her to eat. Since then, expectant mothers have been more happily eating for two within the recommended range of 25 to 35 pounds. Few doctors bat an eye if a woman gains more than 40 pounds. Most doctors now say that the amount women should gain depends on her pre-pregnancy body mass index, with thin women needing to gain more than heavy ones.

In addition to consuming more calories, pregnant women are also generally healthier than they used to be. They pop vitamins and folic acid, and they are avoiding alcohol, tobacco, and even caffeine. To glean how much of a shift in behavior this all is, crack the spine of a dusty guidebook for pregnancy called *Safe Convoy*, published in 1944. The book says there is no scientific reason for a moderate smoker to stop when she is expecting, because to quit "at that time may do more harm than good by upsetting the nerves. A good rule for smokers is 'less than a pack a day.'" In an equally startling interview on *Face the Nation* in 1971, the chairman of the board of Philip Morris, confronted with evidence that smoking in pregnancy leads to low birth weight, famously said: "Some women would prefer having smaller babies."

While the good news is that the weight increase is likely because women are healthier during pregnancy—excluding diabetes from the discussion—the bad news is that the birth canal is not getting larger, because there is not enough genetic variation in the mating pool for that to happen. And so the sudden increase in larger babies has contributed to the tripling of cesareans during the same time period.

If doctors could accurately predict cephalopelvic disproportion (CPD), many long and painful labors might be avoided. Obstetricians once considered large parental shoe size to be the best indicator for CPD. Now they say that if both parents have large heads in relation to their height, chances are good the baby's head will be larger than its mother's pelvis will allow. Armed with that information, an obstetrician might just recommend surgically removing the baby.

Continuing on this trajectory of producing larger and larger babies may eventually have other evolutionary consequences, in which twins and premature births are actually advantageous. Think about this: With twins, while the total weight of the fetuses may be greater than a single baby, they generally are each smaller than one child in utero might be, allowing the mother to birth each of these smaller babies more easily than one large one. A single large fetus might run out of room in the womb before it reaches full development. A premature birth, in that situation, may well be an adaptation to a problem.

More research on that interesting possibility isn't really feasible, however, because modern medicine so quickly turns to the knife. Doctors are easily bypassing the possibility of CPD by performing cesareans. In early 2005, another English woman, a hotel chef married to a fishmonger, gave birth two weeks early to a boy nicknamed Mighty Joe. He weighed 13 pounds, 13 ounces. Mother Sara Griffin, whose diet consisted not of Big Macs but of mussels, cockles, and all sorts of seafood during the pregnancy, had an emergency cesarean after an exhausting seventeen-hour labor. "As soon as I came round from the anesthetic, one of the nurses told me he was the biggest baby that had ever been born there," said Griffin, who is 5 feet, 8 inches. "I was gobsmacked. Thank God for anesthetics."

Is Sara Griffin's story a harbinger of where birth is headed? For an answer, I turned to Professor Lovejoy again, hoping he could explain if there's a way to exit this loop of having large babies and needing cesareans.

"How will this story end?" I asked him.

"Given the rate of technology, one hundred years from now no one will be giving birth. We'll make children up from artificially conceived fetuses, all done technologically," he said mischievously. "What people don't realize today is the explosive advancement of technology that can override evolution. We override evolution to make better tomatoes. There's no reason we can't override evolution to make better humans."

And so the pelvis, obstetrically speaking, could be made obsolete.

It's clear that survival of mother and child depends on many things, from pelvis shape and head size to the position of the baby and physical abnormalities. And it seems evident that evolution's legacy and modern life seem to be increasingly at odds. But the situation is far from hopeless. While a woman's labor may take longer than a monkey's or hurt more than a polar bear's, human birth does succeed in the vast majority of cases. There are 6.5 billion people on this planet to prove the point.

The missing link in all this modern-day success may be the midwife. Although Lucy's own brain might not have been developed enough to make her fear birth and seek help—we just don't know—eventually women came to rely on having companionship to guide them through it. These helpers became the human solution for overriding nature's glitches.

2 MIDWIVES THROUGHOUT TIME

EVERY CULTURE HAS had a system of midwifery, usually informal, with mothers, grandmothers, neighbors, or extended members of the tribe helping women through birth. Brigham Young, the legendary polygamist leader of the Mormon Church, had one of his wives help many of his other wives through their deliveries. Midwives of old—just like their modern counterparts—would tell the mother when to push, rest, or walk. They would use their hands to turn breeches, stimulate the newborn's breathing, unwind the cord from the baby's neck. They offered mothers encouragement, a massage, or a salve, as well as suggestions for position changes to facilitate the birth.

Two centuries ago, midwives were major figures in their communities. They welcomed new life, ushered out the old, and took care of practically everyone in between, sometimes even tending to the health of domesticated animals. They secretly harbored unwed mothers, performed abortions, baptized babies by squirting anointed water in utero, prepared the dead for burial, served as pediatrician during the baby's first year, and looked after the sick using herbal or folk remedies. Some oversaw sanitary conditions at local brothels. Others testified at trials about whether a child had died before or after birth. Midwives vouched for the paternity of the newborn and recorded the baby's birth for local authorities. They probed females about to be married to make sure

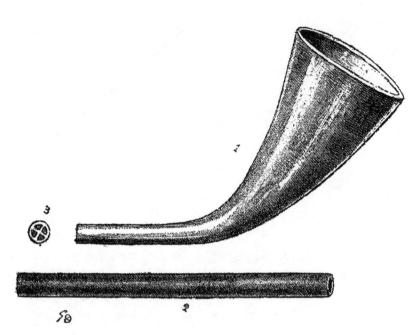

Seventeenth-century midwifery syringe for baptism in utero. (Courtesy the
Wellcome Library)

they would be "fruitful" and diagnosed pregnancy and virginity,
although not always correctly.

They performed all these duties often for little pay. European midwives were occasionally referred to as "grace wives" because mothers presented them with gifts, or grace, a form of
thanks that did not involve currency. Sometimes the midwife's
job of catching a baby in her apron was performed in exchange
for food, clothes, animals, a jug of molasses, or the promise of a
service provided in return. Some villages, including those in the
Lorraine province of France, elected their midwives and gave
them a salary, just like shepherds, considering their services to
be indispensable to the community's welfare.

In 1600, in New Amsterdam, now Manhattan, the town
council voted to name Hellegond Joris official midwife, with an

annual salary of one hundred guilders, the equivalent of about four hundred dollars. For those midwives who were paid by the birth, the fee frequently was better if she delivered a male heir. The delivery of a dead child—even if the fetus died in utero—could mean a smaller fee or no pay at all. If the child was deformed, the midwife might pay with her own life out of suspicion she had caused the aberration.

Midwife, from the Old English, literally means *"with woman."* And that's a very apt description of the role. Midwives were always women, for propriety's sake, but also because they had personal experience with birth. Often, being a grandmother was the only credential a midwife had—or needed—in the millennia before the role was professionalized and doctors emerged. In many languages, *midwife* is the same word as *grandmother.* In Jamaica, regardless of whether the midwife is a blood relative, she's *nana;* in Japan, where midwives still deliver almost all the babies born in hospitals, she's *samba,* or granny, a term of affection. The French call a midwife *sage-femme,* or wise woman. In ancient Greece, law mandated that midwives had to have sons or daughters of their own and be postmenopausal; having stopped bearing children, she would have the time and knowledge to help others. Likewise, a Dublin hospital that began formally training midwives in 1774 considered only those applicants who were married mothers between thirty and forty years old, an age range that would have included those at the tail end of their own reproductive cycles who were still fit and energetic enough to assist during the birth and the days after.

Given humanity's long dependence on midwives, and the comfort and safety they can provide, one would think these women would still reign today. But that is not the case. In my own family, nearly two dozen of us spread among four generations were unilaterally delivered by obstetricians. Yet if things had been different, if midwives had attended all of our births, would generation after generation of my family's maternity stories have been so dramatically unpleasant?

Midwifery through the ages has had more ups and downs than those uterine contraction profiles printed out from tocodynamometers beside a modern hospital bed. Consider the story of Sarah Stone. Stone was a busy and respected midwife in the English countryside in the early 1700s who delivered almost three hundred babies a year. Late one rain-swept night, she received word that a tanner's wife was in labor. Stone grabbed her cloak and headed out. But the tanner's home was eight miles away and by the time she arrived, the baby already had been born. Its slippery body had been caught by another midwife, who insisted everything was fine and tried to turn Stone away. Stone refused to leave, climbed the stairs, and discovered the baby had one eye out, much of its facial skin torn off, and the upper lip shredded from the jawbone.

"How did the child's face become so miserably hurt?" Stone asked the other midwife.

"The mother fell down two days before she was in travail," the midwife replied evasively.

"I am sensible enough," Stone snapped, to know "that the child came head foremost, but the face presented to the birth; and the damage the child received was from your fingers."

The midwife had no defense. More than likely, she also had no training and no license and was so poor that she rushed the birth in order to collect the delivery fee before Stone could intervene. The experience infuriated Stone, who, as an author and outstanding practitioner, was fighting to keep the profession respectable in the face of its worsening reputation. She did not succeed. At least not in her lifetime.

Until early last century, midwives rarely had any formal education. This was because many societies discouraged or even banned women from attending schools or learning to read. As such, midwives usually were self-taught, learning as those around them called for help, or through apprenticeships. If a midwife could read, she may have learned a few standard techniques from *The Byrth of Mankynde*, the first English-language text on the subject, originally published by a man in England in 1540. But not all written information was helpful. In the seventeenth century, Jane Sharp, the first British midwife to write a book about pregnancy and birth, included astrological charts in her 1671 text, *The Midwife's Book*. In it, she explained how to hold a stone "near the privy parts" to draw out the baby or, if that didn't work, to knit coriander seeds with clean linen cloth held at the laboring woman's left thigh. Sharp also recommended a fresh sheepskin on the back of a sore new mother or a bloody hare skin on her belly.

Until the nineteenth century, regardless of whether the local midwife was capable or not, there were no practical alternatives for the vast majority of women giving birth, so the profession persevered. Ultimately, however, midwives would be impotent in fighting the vicious attacks from formalized medicine in the late nineteenth and early twentieth centuries, when freshly minted male doctors, desperate for customers, began attending births. These physicians urged women to forget about personal modesty, promising them pain relief and safer deliveries. They also reminded soon-to-be mothers how "ignorant" and "dirty" midwives were by publicizing examples of bungled births. Their campaign was remarkably successful.

In 1910, midwives were delivering only half of all American babies; the women they helped were mostly blacks and immigrants—those who had little choice or did not want a doctor. By 1930, midwife-attended births had dwindled to 15 percent and were primarily in the South, where doctors were few and far between. By 1973, midwives were handling less than 1 percent of U.S. deliveries.

Yet, just when it looked as if midwives might become extinct, the natural childbirth movement blossomed, celebrating midwifery for its old-fashioned gentleness and commonsense approach. Newly liberated women didn't necessarily want male doctors during their labor and delivery, and they wanted to be conscious during birth, something few doctors allowed. So once again, women called for midwives. No longer disparaged, the revived profession now attends about 10 percent of all vaginal births in the United States, a rate that is expected to rise.

VERY SUPERSTITIOUS

Since ancient times, women have relied on wives' tales, icons, and rituals to make sense of pregnancy and birth, to determine everything from the baby's sex to its due date. Many of these folk practices were ingrained in a midwife's job. An Irish midwife might have burned grass and frankincense on a red stone so as to fumigate the woman to prepare her for conception. Squatting over smoke, however, may have been preferable to having a garlic clove suppository, a fertility aid that German midwives prescribed.

Midwives gave laboring women birthing beads, goddess idols, eagle stones (a hollow rock filled with pebbles), flint, amber, or emeralds, as charms for healthy outcomes. They placed a dried rose of Jericho in a bowl of water and waited for it to slowly open, just as the woman was expected to.

Medieval midwives sometimes kept one fingernail long and sharp in order to puncture a pregnant woman's amniotic sac. This talon-like nail came to be a sign of a witch, still evident in cartoonish Halloween depictions today. Another popular early method for a midwife to break the waters was rubbing a crystal of salt on the amniotic sac. She could administer ergot, a fungus that lives on rye, to fire up contractions or use the poisonous belladonna flower, a relaxant, to slow things down. In later years, she might carry string and a knife to cut the cord, perhaps a vial of holy water, some herbs and salves.

Though it was an age of great superstition, church leaders began to grow uncomfortable with a midwife's chants, potions, pagan customs, and late-night darting from house to house. In times of ignorance, the fingers of midwives seemed to mingle with unknown forces, delivering babies that were either rosy or livid, wailing or silent, perfect or deformed. God was supposed to be responsible for controlling life and death—not midwives.

In 1486 two German Dominican monks scratched their ink-dipped quills over parchment to produce the *Malleus maleficarum.* Their tome, which translates as *The Hammer of Witches,* was a practical guide to witch hunting, explaining how to find potential witches. On that point, the *Malleus maleficarum* was strident: "No one does more harm to the Catholic faith than midwives."

Britain executed its first witch in 1479; another thirty thousand were put to death by 1736, when criminal laws against the craft finally were repealed. Across Europe between 1560 and 1660 as many as two hundred thousand "witches" were tried, a huge number considering the relatively small population of the area at the time. About half of those tried were killed, including thirty thousand in Germany (though there were no executions on Sundays). Countless others were executed in Italy, Switzerland, and France (four hundred in a single day in Toulouse). Sometimes the witch hunts were small in scope; other times they were large-scale mob scenes. In 1585, two German villages were left with one female inhabitant each. Witch hunting was so culturally ingrained that if a midwife arrived at the scene of a birth in eastern England more quickly than expected, she ran the risk of being accused of riding her broom there.

No one knows how many of these so-called witches were midwives, but those working women were especially vulnerable to suspicion because they fit the target profile. Witch hunters believed that single women, particularly widows, would be more likely to seek out the devil, because, without a man in their lives, such women needed Lucifer's help just to get by. As well, witches were known to be outspoken and independent. Of course, many midwives, by virtue of being older women who worked for a living, likely were outspoken, independent widows. Also, their role as village healer often involved them in seemingly mysterious occurrences—food that spoiled, men who caught fevers, and babies born with defects. Others aroused suspicion by selling placentas and amniotic membranes for potions or good luck.

In sixteenth-century England, in an attempt to cleanse the profession of alleged sorcerers, authorities began to require midwives to have licenses, issued by the church. The church was, remarkably, less concerned with the applicant's abilities than her promises to shun witchcraft and to immediately baptize a fragile baby, sometimes even before it was born.

Eleanor Pead received one such license after standing before the archbishop of Canterbury in 1567. Her hand on a Bible, Pead pledged that she would help rich and poor through labor, name the baby's rightful father, properly bury stillborn babies, and

> not use any kind of sorcery or incantation in the time of the travail of any woman; and that I will not destroy the child born of any woman, not cut, nor pull off the head thereof, or otherwise dismember or hurt the same, or suffer it to be hurt or dismembered by any manner of way or means. Also . . . at the ministration of the sacrament of baptism in the time of necessity, I will use apt and accustomed words of the same sacrament—that is to say, these words following, or the like in effect: I christen thee in the name of the Father, the Son, and the Holy Ghost, and none other profane words.

In addition to taking the oath, she had to provide recommendations about her skill from women who had relied on her in the past, as well as proof that she was a member of the Church of England. She paid the church about eighteen shillings for the license.

By the 1600s, English pilgrims were disembarking in Colonial America, which desperately needed midwives to maintain a vulnerable but expanding population. When Mary Dyer went into labor in Boston, well-known midwife Jane Hawkins was there to catch the baby, a deformed headless stillborn referred to simply as a "monster." Hawkins was accused of being a witch. In 1638, magistrates forbade her from practicing. Three years later she was forced out of the colony.

Despite Hawkins's banishment, witch hunting was still rare in the settlements, which frequently offered free housing to a midwife if, in return, "she doth not refuse when called to it." The colonists deemed midwifery to be so important that midwives were allowed to ride ferries for free and pass over toll bridges without paying. Tombstones and eulogies from the period show just how valued a midwife's work was. When midwife Ann Eliot died in Roxbury, Massachusetts, in 1687, the public built a tomb and inscribed upon it: "She was thus honored for the great service she hath done this town." When a midwife in Guilford, Connecticut, was eulogized, the pastor said glowingly, "She knew when to exert herself vigorously and also when it was her strength to sit still."

Yet midwives in America would lose their professional edge to a much greater degree and far more quickly than their European counterparts did. In the decades after Jane Hawkins was run out of the colony, Cotton Mather, the famous Massachusetts minister, began to preach that "no midwives can do what Angels can." Mather's message, that birth was in God's hands, effectively helped women to stop thinking that midwives had special powers. Meanwhile, the medical profession hurried to keep pace with the needs of a growing and sprawling population. By the 1750s, although there were no medical schools in America, men were returning from Europe trained as doctors and aggressively searching for wealthy pregnant women willing to pay their much higher birthing fees. The competition between physicians and midwives became so intense that the female attendants were pressed to take out newspaper ads.

MIDWIVES VERSUS MEN

In 1601, when Marie de' Medici, the Queen of France, chose Louise Bourgeois as her midwife, the decision triggered a chain of events that would come to symbolize the debate over who was most qualified to deliver a child—man or woman.

Because she delivered the queen of a male heir—France's first in more than eighty years—Bourgeois became a luminary in great demand among the upper crust of Parisian society. She chronicled her most unusual cases in an ambitious 1609 book, the first ever by a midwife, entitled *Observations diverses sur la sterilité perte de fruict foecondité accouchements et maladies des femmes et enfants nouveaux naiz*—Observations about sterility, loss of the fertilized ovum, fecundity and childbirth and female and newborn diseases.

The book explained her philosophy that a midwife was like a pilot at sea keeping the crew safe in a storm. The tome detailed how to induce labor if a woman's pelvis was too small to pass a full-term fetus; what to do if the umbilical cord emerged before the baby (a potentially deadly situation); and how to deliver a child that perilously presented face-first. The work set out to promote ethical and practical standards—benchmarks for other midwives to follow. But not all were comfortable with the midwife's newfound fame.

Early in her career Bourgeois had ingratiated herself with male surgeons, needing their help to gain respect from and access to their wealthy clients. (Because male surgeons were the only ones allowed to use forceps during births, they commanded high fees.) Once Bourgeois became a famous midwife, however, she began publicly attacking surgeons for their meddlesome mistakes that complicated what should have been normal births. Her condemnations made them seethe.

In 1627, Bourgeois was called to the first delivery of the young Duchess of Orleans, the wealthiest heiress in France. The child was a girl, not an heir, and the duchess died nine days later. Marie de' Medici, who was still queen, was furious and called for an autopsy. A horde of surgeons pounced to comply with her wishes. They found that the duchess had peritonitis, an infection they said was caused by a small piece of hardened placenta left inside the uterus, something Bourgeois should have noticed after inspecting the afterbirth.

Bourgeois denied the accusation and printed a public letter that said the duchess had "cancer in the lower parts of the abdomen" and accused the examiners of trying to blame and discredit her with this fabricated idea about peritonitis. She was forced to retire early—a genteel punishment compared with the fiery deaths some earlier midwives faced.

Bourgeois's fate foreshadowed what would happen to other midwives, in both Europe and America, as doctors encroached on their livelihood. One typical case occurred in 1793, on the rugged Maine coast, where midwife Martha Ballard had been delivering babies for nearly a decade with an outstanding record for both mother and child. On this occasion, she had been up all night with the pregnant young bride Hannah Sewall. Although Ballard knew that patience was called for, especially since first labors can take more than a day, Sewall's nervous husband felt that something should be done. He called in a twenty-four-year-old male doctor, Ben Page, who was taking advantage of a local baby boomlet to elbow his way into Ballard's practice, something she fumed about in her diary. Page—who charged six dollars per delivery compared with Ballard's two dollars—"gave my patient 20 drops of Laudanum which put her into such a stupor her pains (which were regular & promising) in a manner stopt till near night when she pukt & they

returned & shee delivered at 7 hour Evening of a son her first Born,"
Ballard wrote in her journal. In another case that Ballard complained
of, Page's inexperience delivering a breech led to a dead baby with
dislocated limbs. Ballard did not have such devastating outcomes.
Only in about 5 percent of her 814 birth cases over twenty-seven
years did she note any sort of complication with a birth. She had a
less than 2 percent stillborn rate, less than 3 percent neonatal death
rate, and less than 1 percent maternal mortality.

It did not matter that Ballard was the better attendant then,
or that her record was better than hospitals and their doctors
would provide. Around the world, female birth attendants, re-
vered throughout time, were being rendered second class.

UPGRADING THE PROFESSION

The trouble was, there were not enough male attendants to replace
midwives, and too few women were ready to trade the old, comfortable maternity system for a new one that involved giving birth
in the presence of a man.

Despite the Bourgeois case culminating in the death of the
Duchess, France, whose population had been depleted by war, disease, and infant mortality, was particularly vexed about this situation. So much so that King Louis XV, who reigned from 1715 to 1774,
believed that his people's future depended on sound midwifery
skills. Rather than create more surgeons, he decided that midwives
should be better trained and took the unusual step of appointing
a national midwife to instruct others in the art of safe deliveries.
Her name was Madame du Coudray.

Du Coudray was young, single, and childless when she set
out to become a midwife, making her both an oddity and a sensation. She traveled across France in the mid-eighteenth century with
a fabric-wrapped handmade birth simulation machine that she had
devised. She taught midwives who, for the most part, did not want

her advice. Regardless, her work and that of the king appears to have paid off. With midwives trained from the Pyrenees to Paris, France's population began increasing sharply.

In America, formal midwife training began in 1848, when a man named Samuel Gregory, shocked that male doctors saw laboring women's private parts, responded by founding the Boston Female Medical College, the first school of its kind in the country. At the time members of the Boston Medical Society attacked Gregory—a bachelor without a medical degree—saying it was he who had unchaste thoughts. Despite that initial criticism, the school remained operational for more than two decades, before finally closing in 1874.

Meanwhile, throughout the late nineteenth century, male doctors cast those waves of immigrant midwives who had come to America as relics of an outmoded European lifestyle. The men also launched public education campaigns promoting the ideas that birth was painful and should be treated like a disease, and that male attendants were best qualified to handle deliveries. These early campaigns were brutally effective. By and large, midwives were left to care for those who could not afford—or did not live near—a doctor.

By 1900, midwifery had lost half its base to doctors. Those still using midwives tended to be immigrants, who trusted other women—just as they had in the old country—and could not pay doctors' higher fees. In 1912, for example, the average mill worker in Lawrence, Massachusetts, earned less than nine dollars per week. A midwife there charged five dollars a birth, often accepting flexible payment or food for services, which might include household help or daily checkups for up to ten days. A physician, on the other hand, never cleaned the kitchen, provided just one or two postpartum visits, and charged double the fee of a midwife, demanding cash payment at the time of delivery.

Yet, despite being the less expensive option, midwives continued to dwindle, in part because of a doctor-led campaign against what was commonly called "the midwife problem." In the 1920s, doctors wrote to popular magazines, blaming midwives for maternal infections and neonatal ophthalmia, blindness caused by the mother's gonorrhea. (Although silver nitrate eyedrops could prevent this, midwives were barred from using the liquid because it was considered a drug.)

Instead of instituting strict certification requirements, which is what happened throughout Europe in the nineteenth and early twentieth centuries, the American medical establishment actually restricted training in an attempt to make midwives go away. States began outlawing the profession. Almost immediately, however, infant mortality increased in some areas. Why? Obstetricians were remarkably poorly trained at delivering babies.

J. Whitridge Williams was a professor of obstetrics at the Johns Hopkins University in Baltimore. In 1912, he sent a questionnaire to 120 medical schools that offered four-year courses in obstetrics. Williams was fishing for data to support his opposition to midwifery and wanted to document how much better educated and equipped doctors were. He did not find what he expected. Professors confessed to him that they were unprepared to teach, unqualified to handle obstetric emergencies, and nearly all said they had inadequate hospital equipment. Most serious of all, Williams discovered that "a large proportion admit that the average practitioner, through his lack of preparation for the practice of obstetrics, may do his patients as much harm as the much-maligned midwife." One professor conceded that he had never seen a live birth before he began teaching. A quarter of the professors said they could not handle a case of ruptured uterus. When asked who was more responsible for spreading infection, professors confessed that doctors were equally to blame as midwives. They even believed that doctors were more likely than a midwife to kill a mother or child.

One would think that such a report would lead Williams to renewed respect for midwives, a decrease in respect for doctors, and some reform of childbirth training. But Williams, a well-known figure in the medical establishment, wielded the information like a sword—and lunged at midwives.

"Why bother about the relatively innocuous midwife," Williams wrote, "when the ignorant doctor causes quite as many absolutely unnecessary deaths? From the nature of things, it is impossible to do away with the physician, but he may be educated in time; while the midwife can eventually be abolished, if necessary. Consequently, we should direct our efforts to reforming the existing practitioner and to changing our methods of training students so as to make the physician of the future reasonably competent."

And so it went.

MODERN MIDWIVES

Not every midwife closed shop, however. In the 1930s, there were still about fifty thousand midwives in the United States, 80 percent of whom were in the South. The rural poor had neither hospitals nor cars nor money to get them to facilities to see a doctor. In truth, these weren't patients white doctors even wanted to deliver. Instead, black women known as grannies delivered the majority of babies, of all races, south of the Mason-Dixon Line up until the 1970s.

The work was often done out of charity, and many of the grannies considered midwifery a spiritual calling. Aunt Quintilla was among them. Her ordinary yet colorful story might have been forgotten if not for a 1930 *Harper's Monthly* article that portrayed her as a curiosity at a time when the rest of the country—at least the northern part—had already migrated toward hospital deliveries with doctors. Drawn to the job by an apparition from God, Quintilla said she ignored Him at first. But God was persistent. His voice came to her again one day when she was washing clothes in a sudsy tub on the back porch. Suddenly, a hand holding a fiery sword pierced through the mounds of bubbles.

"Quintilla, why ain't you obeyed de call?" the voice said.

Quintilla rushed into the yard jumping and screaming, pulling on her hair.

"I'se got de call! I'se got de call," she shouted.

The first slave boat that had arrived in America in 1619 brought with it the West African midwifery ways. Like their European counterparts, these grannies embraced folk traditions and used minerals, plants, and herbs for healing. For a case of childbed fever, grannies might have tied a piece of hog's meat around the mother's neck and dusted it with pepper. For a slow labor, they might have thrown hen feathers on coals beneath a bed, hung a bear-tooth necklace on the woman, or made her wear her husband's clothes.

Throughout the 1930s, Quintilla, who lived in Virginia, used these ancient rites in combination with modern antiseptic techniques taught by the local health board. The health boards also verified permits, tracked ages and length of service, and inspected birth bags, which in addition to the standard fare, might also include such things as "a vial of April snow water" for the newborn's eyes.

The granny traditions were among the last to die in contemporary times, outlawed in Alabama, for example, in 1976. There are several reasons grannies, as a profession, endured longer than midwives elsewhere in the United States: They served a disenfranchised population that no one else wanted to serve, and they did it well. Some practiced for forty years without losing a mother or child.

Tucked away in the hills of Appalachia was another disenfranchised and segregated population, poor whites, with few services and big families. Out of those desperate circumstances something remarkable emerged.

In 1912, the U.S. government established the Children's Bureau to look into, among other things, why 124 babies per 1,000 live births were dying nationwide, a rate of more than 12 percent. The investigation found that many women were often sick going into pregnancy and did not get proper care in the months before the birth. The report ultimately led to the call for public health nurses to provide prenatal care. But there was still a problem. Few public health nurses were trained in pregnancy and birth—that was a midwife's job.

Enter Mary Breckinridge, whose two children had died when they were very young. Divorced and alone, Breckinridge was a rare upper-class woman who had been trained as a nurse. She also happened to be looking for a cause. In the summer of 1923, she rode seven hundred miles on horseback through the hills of Appalachia, offering aid to fourteen-year-olds who were still picking corn in the fields when they were nine months pregnant. As well, Breckinridge met with dozens of midwives, who smoked pipes and practiced their own brand of deliveries, from feeding tea made of soot to women in labor, to placing an ax, edge up, under their beds to facilitate birth.

Breckinridge realized that she needed her own midwifery skills, in addition to her nursing degree. But in America, nurses were not midwives. In Britain they were both—trained nurses with additional expertise in delivering babies. And so Breckinridge went to the U.K. to become one of the first Americans trained as a nurse-midwife. She brought her new skills back to the United States, establishing, in 1925, in the remote mountains of Kentucky, what would become the Frontier Nursing Service. Breckinridge did not recruit American women. She couldn't. Most states were by then eliminating midwifery training. So she imported nurse-midwives from England and Scotland. They wore trousers and sheepskin coats, rode horseback, carried snakebite serum in their saddlebags, and attended the ever growing number of births in that area.

The Frontier Nursing Service's outcomes were outstanding. By 1951, the nurse-midwives had delivered 8,596 babies. Though they dealt with breeches, toxemias, and hemorrhages, the staff, which included only one doctor, used forceps only fifty times, and performed only forty cesareans. Breckinridge said the good results had to do in part with the facts that the pregnant women had been breast-fed themselves and exposed to sunshine (rickets was rare) and the population was homogenous, so that no one had to pull "a [large] Mediterranean head through a [narrow] Nordic pelvis."

From that remote Appalachian outpost, the modern nurse-midwifery concept began to spread. By 1931, the Maternity Center Association established America's first nurse-midwifery program in New York City. Columbia-Presbyterian hospital, also in New York, launched a nurse-midwifery program in 1955, becoming the country's first hospital to offer nurses extra obstetrical training.

By 1971, when the American College of Obstetricians and Gynecologists finally approved nurse-midwifery for uncomplicated maternity cases, there were about twelve hundred certified practitioners in the United States. Four years later nurse-midwives could practice in almost every state. There was good reason for the medical establishment to accept nurse-midwives: As baby boomers began to reproduce, the birthrate outstripped the number of obstetricians. Meanwhile, women, empowered by the liberation movement, were looking for a kinder, gentler birth experience, one that did not involve obstetricians or even hospitals.

A new generation, preferring to give birth at home, often still had to rely on uncertified help—women who were willing to commit a misdemeanor to catch the baby. Raven Lang is a prime— and somewhat famous—example of how traditional home-birth midwifery was reinvented as part of the counterculture revolution. Lang had been an art teacher. Her only training in midwifery was in tending a herd of fertile goats and the traumatic birth of her son, in 1968, in a hospital near San Francisco.

"I didn't think I was going to be a guinea pig," she said, in an interview. "I was only in [the hospital] four hours before my baby was born. I must have had fifty internal exams. They were all residents and interns. It was every ten minutes, and every ten minutes it was somebody new." At the time Lang was twenty-five, a dancer who wanted to walk around during labor. They made her stay in bed.

"At that point," she said, "you're pretty vulnerable. You don't know what to expect not only from labor, but from the protocols of the hospital. So I was obedient, so to speak. During the delivery they gave me an episioproctotomy, a cut in the perineum that goes through the anterior part of the anal sphincter. The side effect is that you can't poop the next day or the next. You can't make love for months without pain, and you can't really pick up a baby without pain. You can't lift things, and you can't sit down on things. There was nothing—not even a nano-thought—that was going to prepare me for that kind of abuse."

California had outlawed midwifery in 1949. Two decades later, young people, especially in the Bay Area, were busily overturning both convention and law, including how birth was handled. This movement produced women such as Lang, who became a "lay" or uncertified midwife credited with spreading the ideology of the home-birth movement of the 1970s. The legendary midwife, Ina May Gaskin, also was called into service during that era. She peeled out of California to proselytize a more spiritual way of life and on her journey began delivering friends' babies in the backs of buses. Gaskin's group morphed into a Tennessee commune known as The Farm, which became a sort of freestanding birth center that still attracts pregnant women from around the world. Gaskin has reached cult-like stature even among professional midwives and doctors. Her technique for delivering babies whose broad shoulders get stuck is to have the mother get down on all fours. This is known as the Gaskin maneuver and is taught today in obstetrical classes.

Raven Lang's entry into midwifery, however, had more to do with her outrage over hospital birth practices than any sort of free-spirited happenstance.

"What we have now," she recalled, "simply didn't exist. We didn't have midwives, we didn't have childbirth educators. We had zip."

Within six months of her baby's arrival, Lang and her family moved south to the bohemian paradise of Santa Cruz. Lang raised goats in the hills, watching them give birth, learning nature's way. One day a woman who lived in a Volkswagen bus and breast-fed her baby in public—a rarity then—met Lang at her home to talk to her about birth.

"She was lactating and I was lactating, and I took to her like a bee to honey," Lang said. "Within the first ten minutes I found out she had had her baby at home."

"What happened when you needed to cut your perineum?" Lang asked the young mother.

"When you have to cut what? What's a perineum? No, we didn't cut it."

"Did it tear?" Lang wanted to know.

"No."

"Let me see your vagina," Lang requested.

A friendship was born.

This young new friend invited Lang to witness a delivery that night.

"It was like a miracle. It was her first child, she was in labor, and I was there for the entire night. In the morning her baby was born. Everything went beautifully."

Shortly thereafter, Lang began teaching birthing classes and served as birth coach for her students. "After [witnessing] thirty-five births somebody asked me if I would attend her, and I attended her as midwife . . . I caught her baby. I was not technically a midwife, but this was a time when people were redefining their social selves. The community was calling me a midwife. Women were attending women with graciousness and letting women be in control," Lang said.

She and a few others established a birth center in a Santa Cruz home in 1970. (This was about the same time Raven Lang ditched her real first name, Patricia.) The free services included prenatal and postpartum care. The center, located in the home of Kate Bowland, thrived. Lang's reputation grew and in 1972, she was called to Canada to open two birth centers. Meanwhile, back home, police were organizing a sting operation against the Santa Cruz facility, where a group of about ten women were working.

When law enforcement raided the center, Bowland called Lang, who was back in town.

"The place is being invaded by police," Bowland said. "They're going through my house with a fine-tooth comb."

"I'll be there, and I'm calling all the papers," Lang told her.

When Lang arrived at the scene, neither the police nor the FBI, looking to take her to jail, recognized her; she evaded arrest. Three others, however, were charged with practicing medicine without a license.

"We knew it was the beginning of what was going to come," Lang recalled.

The California Court of Appeals eventually ruled on the case, declaring that "pregnancy and childbirth are not diseases but rather normal physiological functions of women." The midwives had not violated any medical codes. But their celebration was short-lived. The state's supreme court issued a ruling prohibiting the practice of midwifery without a certificate, forcing many of these renegades into the uncomfortable position of joining the establishment by becoming certified nurse-midwives.

Lang was considered a "lay midwife," someone working without a license or formal midwifery education. No one knows precisely how many lay midwives remain in the United States because they are still illegal, but one estimate is that there are more than two thousand of them attending home births and being paid out of pocket by clients.

The largest accepted designation by far is the nurse-midwife, who almost always works in a hospital. There are about six thousand practicing in America today, and consumer demand for them is rising. But the profession is aging. Just look in any ballroom at a midwifery convention and you will see chairs filled with gray-haired, Birkenstock-wearing women who were clearly drawn into the field during a wave of passion in the 1970s. They are an earnest bunch that gets teary when they tell each other dramatic birth stories, and they wear cheeky T-shirts in their off hours saying "At your cervix." They have become the defenders of birth as a "normal" process. They talk lovingly about breast-feeding and recount stories of women who have had orgasms during the pushing phase of a drug-free birth.

But after all these years, despite the growing body of evidence that they provide excellent birth outcomes, midwives are still fighting the same battles for respect and market share. In the past, arguments against midwives have always focused on safety, an issue central to every mother's mind. By withholding the proper licensing and education of midwives, governments paradoxically made a woman's decision about who would attend her birth more complicated and potentially even lethal. It took the power of the counterculture revolution and the force of the women's movement to push back on the outdated stereotypes, to call for reform, and to help some women understand why midwives are better than doctors for attending low-risk births.

The statistics support their claims. In America, those women attended by midwives ultimately have lower cesarean rates, fewer interventions such as labor induction and episiotomies, and lower infant mortality, than those attended by doctors. The same holds true abroad. In the Netherlands, where midwives attend nearly half of all births, the country's maternal mortality rate is even lower than America's, with 16 deaths per 100,000 births compared to our 17 per 100,000. About 30 percent of Dutch births occur at home, quite safely, a trend driven by cultural ideals about family life. The little-known truth is that having a baby at home with a midwife, even in the United States, regularly produces better outcomes than delivering in a hospital. A study by Eugene Declercq at the Boston University School of Public Health looked at more than eighty thousand home births in the United States between 1989 and 1992. The mothers tended to be older and to have had less prenatal care. In essence, these women had higher-risk pregnancies. But the outcomes were no worse than all those "normal" hospital deliveries, according to the study.

Midwives seem to make sense. They can provide excellent care. They charge less than doctors. And their services often continue after the birth. Yet, although more women may be realizing this, the vast majority of us still do the same things at the first twinge of labor. Call the OB. Lumber to the car. Drive the practiced route—straight to the hospital.

3 THE HUT, THE HOME, AND THE HOSPITAL

BABIES HAVE BEEN born just about everywhere—farm fields, parking lots, traffic-stalled taxicabs, airplanes, subways, and high school bathrooms on prom night. But throughout history, most births have occurred in more carefully selected locations: On the Kapingamarangi atoll in Micronesia, laboring women sought shallow water at the ocean's edge. Ancient Egyptians had their babies in special buildings, the walls decorated with depictions of Isis and Pacht, the goddess and god of childbirth. Poor French women delivered in wards called the *salle sauvage,* or savage room. And in the antebellum American South, although plantation masters valued slave women as "breeders," their social status still relegated them to give birth near—or in—horse stalls, where babies often contracted tetanus from the manure. Still, other women living freely in the countryside chose to give birth in the stables. In the Auvergne region of France, for example, doing so was common practice in the 1800s, and the custom persisted elsewhere in Europe into the twentieth century for understandable reasons: If the house was small and there were lots of other children around, a woman might feel more comfortable moaning in the barn, and she later wouldn't have to clean up fluids that were considered impure and corrosive.

Some cultures were quite specific in their beliefs about how polluting birth could be. The Maori and the Japanese banned laboring women from the house to keep out the mess, and with it, evil spirits. In parts of China, women delivered in huts that were set on fire after the lying-in period. The Inuits built huts made of snow or skins, where women gave birth alone. At least, that was their custom until the Canadian government, in the 1970s, ordered all pregnant women evacuated from their homes and flown eight hours south, well before their due dates, to deliver in a proper hospital, far, far away from their families.

Of course, some babies have been born in places that were neither accidental nor deliberate, but unavoidable—on covered wagons crossing the North American plains, on the *Mayflower* (the boy was named Oceanus), in prisons and concentration camps.

But throughout most of history, until about a hundred years ago, almost all women gave birth at home, surrounded by midwife, friends, and family. In England, these helpers were assembled by the father, after knocking door to door, or "nidgeting," throughout the village. In sixteenth-century France, the task of locating the *sage-femme* was simpler because there would have been a sign with symbols, such as a woman holding a baby, or a cradle marked with a *fleur-de-lis*, hanging outside her house. Once in attendance, these women would assist not just in the birth, but in taking care of mother and baby postpartum, from dressing the infant to changing the bed linens, to feeding the husband, knowing such favors would be returned.

Birth was a time for celebrating motherhood; it was also a social event. In Europe and early America, there would be so much chattering and sharing of information during labor that these "God-sibs," or sisters-in-God, would become the basis for the word *gossip*. It's no wonder that Louis XIV of France took the unusual step of employing a man to deliver his mistress, Louise de la Valliere; surely a midwife would not keep the bastard's birth a secret.

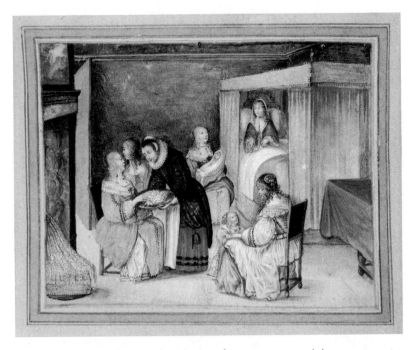

A seventeenth-century Dutch painting shows a woman giving sweetmeats to the gossips. (Courtesy the Wellcome Library)

These women didn't just mill around and make noise. They quickly readied the house for the event, breaking out "childbed linen," or heirloom layette, passed down generation to generation, or given as wedding presents. Birth would take place on older soft linen or on rags in "the borning room," often an area near the central fire that was partitioned off for privacy and to protect the mother and baby from drafts. Curtains were drawn; sometimes even the keyholes were stuffed to exclude outside air, evil spirits, and prying eyes from penetrating the space. The borning room also might be the master bedroom, where mother and child could stay throughout the lying-in period—a time of rest while her help remained at the house. Another popular place to give birth at home was in front of the kitchen hearth, perhaps on a tuft of straw, functioning the same way a "splash mat" works on hospital beds today. When the birth was over, the midwife could throw the straw into the fire and the mess was gone. The words "in the straw" became a colloquialism to describe a woman having a baby.

In most cases, the man of the house would light the fire and leave, keeping company with the other men whose wives had left them to attend the birth. For some women, an after-nurse would arrive to cook and clean when the neighborhood circle and midwife left. Before that happened the gossips would throw a feast, sometimes called a "groaning party," named with a nod to both the sounds of labor and those of the stuffed women after they ate.

Although home births continued through the end of the nineteenth century, the atmosphere began to change as male physicians, rather than midwives, arrived to attend the births. Occasionally, especially during the early years of this remarkable transition, a midwife and doctor both would be at the house, arguing over how to best treat the woman. The gossips, who may have had enough children between them to fill a classroom, might have also stood around the bed, participating in the debate.

Physicians, not surprisingly, were anxious to evict these helpers from the home. In one 1887 manual for women, the author, a physician, instructs the mother-to-be to carefully choose and limit who would be by her bed supporting her. "Many attendants are not only unnecessary but injurious," Dr. P. B. Saur wrote in *Maternity: A Book for Every Wife and Mother*. "They excite and flurry the patient, they cause noise and confusion and rob the air of its purity. One lady friend, besides the doctor and the nurse, is all that's needed. In making the selection of a friend, care should be taken that she is the mother of a family, that she is kind-hearted and self-possessed, and of a cheerful turn of mind. All chatterers, croakers, and putterers ought, at these times, to be carefully excluded from the room. No conversation of a depressing character should for one moment be allowed."

Aside from choosing attendants, the pregnant woman also had to arrange the house and sometimes even gather her own supplies, whether it was brandy to be used as an anesthetic, string and scissors to tie and cut the umbilical cord, or a pot of lard to massage the perineum.

These preparations by the mother, and group care by the gossips, would eventually be replaced by a more systematic, institutional lying-in. It was not, at least early on, a positive change.

HOSPITALS

In the eighteenth century, industrialization in Europe and America created conditions that bred disease and injury, forcing governments to open hospitals in response. These buildings, and others devoted solely to helping expectant mothers, were places where only the indigent or unmarried pregnant women checked in. You would not find any self-respecting middle-class women in these hospitals. They still gave birth at home.

For those who were admitted to these early wards, the care was free, but the services came with a price: Often, women were used as obstetrical guinea pigs. The first experiments for artificially inducing labor were conducted on charity cases in England. Moreover, the facilities in which they were treated were horrid. Paris's venerable Hotel Dieu, one of the world's first obstetric teaching clinics, was so crowded in its early years that its twelve hundred large beds held as many as six patients at a time, perhaps placing a laboring woman side-by-side with a consumptive child. The floors were covered with straw and infested with vermin. There was no ventilation.

Yet despite how horrible these facilities were, women with no other choice literally lined up for admittance. At the Rotunda in Dublin, the British Isles' first lying-in hospital, established in 1745, women had to apply for a labor bed. The staff instructed expectant mothers to bring clean clothes for themselves and their babies; they also had to be free of lice and venereal disease. The Rotunda was so overwhelmed with patients that women there also shared beds—although just with each other—during their seven-day stay. The hospital did not have hot running water until the late nineteenth century. Hot baths were given only upon admittance (lest the incoming spread filth to others), though most women probably would have preferred one after delivering.

Because of the population they served, many early maternity hospitals operated much like reform schools. In the mid-1700s, the British Lying-In charity hospital expressly prohibited swearing, smoking, drinking gin, and playing cards or dice. The facility expelled women for having lice, being rude, or, understandably, pretending to be pregnant. Patients' waking, eating, and sleeping were scheduled events, and women could not visit friends in other wards. On top of all that, staff tried to correct patients' bad behavior with sermons and demonstrations. Before they left the hospital, new mothers had to "give thanks," an exit interview of sorts in which the staff quizzed them about their stay and elicited complaints about anything from bad food to bedbugs or negligent staff. The hospital hoped these debriefings would help them fix any problems before benefactors heard about them and stopped offering donations.

Early American maternity wards were equally wretched places, mostly serving poor immigrants in big cities. Mary Connor, a housekeeper, was a thirty-one-year-old unwed Irish woman living in New York in 1860 when she checked herself in to that city's first lying-in facility, at Bellevue Hospital, for the last month of her pregnancy—or confinement, as she would have called it. Her delivery there was horrific. Connor slipped in and out of consciousness. Patients lying a few feet away from her finally called a nurse, who summoned the doctor, Alexander Hadden, who inquired of the problem.

"She stated she thought her child was born. I immediately examined and found the child beneath the hips of the mother, in a lifeless condition, and mutilated, apparently by rats. In the position in which the child was, life could have existed but a few moments," Hadden recalled.

Being imperiled by rats was not the worst of what could befall a pregnant woman in the hospital. When Bridget Logan, an unmarried sixteen-year-old, checked herself in to Boston Lying-In Hospital, in 1883, to await the birth of her baby, she, and all others admitted there, had a 50 percent chance of contracting childbed fever—also called puerperal sepsis—an infection that doctors spread by not washing their hands before a vaginal exam. In an outbreak the year Logan gave birth, 75 percent of the new mothers at that hospital became infected with the fever; 20 percent were killed by it.

On a cold January evening, Logan gave birth to a baby weighing less than six pounds. After the delivery, doctors gave her a standard preventive douche of weak carbolic acid, which they believed helped ward off infection. They did the same the next day. Rather than helping her, however, the douche probably forced the deadly bacteria further into her womb. By the second night, she had contracted the infection. Doctors responded by giving her an "irrigation of the uterus with permanganate of potash" followed by quinine the next day. After a seemingly endless cycle of quinine and douches, she grew feverish. She had ringing in her ears. Her thoughts became nonsensical. Her belly was distended and extremely painful. She vomited and hallucinated, believing other patients were talking about her and trying to kill her. At one point, when the nurse left the room, Logan escaped from the hospital. When she was caught, the staff dragged her back in restraints and gave her a sedative. And then she died.

Logan would have been just another victim if it were not for this depressing statistic: She was the youngest of the fifty women who died of childbed fever at the hospital in a five-year span, during which five hundred had been stricken with the infection.

Childbed fever was just as prevalent in Europe. Because government regulations there required autopsies on mothers who died of the fever, physicians and medical students, who practiced obstetric exams on cadavers, created a devastating cycle by going from the autopsy slab—where decomposing bits of the body would stick under their fingernails and in the creases of their skin—to the delivery table, where they would perform internal exams to check for dilation or descent. At no time in between did they wash their hands. They did not know they should. Louis Pasteur's theory that living microbes, not spontaneous generation, caused putrification did not emerge until the 1860s, the same decade that Joseph Lister's new principles of antisepsis were first applied.

Unhygienic doctors (they also worked in their street clothes) increased the chances during each exam that the mother would be infected with the deadly Group A hemolytic streptococcus, the same germ that causes scarlet fever. The bacteria would travel from his fingers, through the woman's cervix, into the bloodstream and sometimes to the unborn child via the placenta. Doctors also spread staphylococcus aureus from one living patient's wound to another, all because of their dirty hands.

Although the infection was more likely to strike disadvantaged women being attended by doctors in the hospital, puerperal sepsis did not discriminate. Midwives, too, occasionally spread the bacteria, though their less frequent internal exams kept the number of their sepsis cases low, and their one-on-one care did not lead to contagions like those at the hospitals. Among puerperal sepsis's more famous victims were Mary Wollstonecraft—one of Britain's first major feminists, who died ten days after delivering her daughter Mary Shelley, the author of *Frankenstein*—and Jane Seymour, the third of Henry VIII's six wives, who became infected during the delivery of her first child.

For millennia, neither midwives nor doctors had any idea what caused puerperal sepsis. Some believed lactating mothers' milk gone astray was the source of the sickness. Leonardo da Vinci, in his famous coitus drawing, depicted a vein connecting the woman's breast to her uterus. The Hotel Dieu, after one of the first documented hospital epidemics of childbed fever, in 1746, also perpetuated the "milk metastasis theory." When the staff dissected these maternal corpses, they saw what they determined to be "clotted milk" clinging to the intestines and other parts of the abdominal cavity. But it wasn't milk at all. It was infected fluid—pus.

Doctors had other theories that blamed the mother for creating her own infection. Dr. John Clarke of London, in a 1793 text on the management of pregnancy and labor, said tight petticoats in early pregnancy caused fecal backups that infected the bloodstream. Another British doctor, Charles White, blamed self-poisoning by a woman's own vaginal fluids. He ordered that women not be confined to beds with dirty linens. And in 1871, a woman, upset because her husband was abroad when she went into labor at the Rotunda, became infected. The head of the hos-

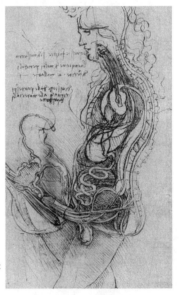

This Leonardo da Vinci drawing, circa 1500, is a mirror image depicting the woman's vein, at left, running from breast to uterus.

pital blamed her fretting, which he said was caused by rumors that other women "were dying like rotten sheep in the hospital." Meanwhile, at the hospital across town where many prostitutes gave birth, reported incidents of puerperal sepsis were rare. That's because those doctors could not be bothered to perform vaginal exams, autopsies, or dissections; the women were not worth the time. The Rotunda's master, however, had another explanation. The prostitutes, he argued, were too depraved to fret.

In America, the president of the newly formed Gynecological Society blamed women's morals for the fever, explaining in 1877 why those having babies in hospitals were more susceptible to the illness. "The majority of patients who seek the lying-in asylums are unmarried," he said. "A poor girl who is ashamed of her condition, who is anxious as to what will become of herself and her offspring, who has been driven away from her place when her state could no longer be concealed, and who has suffered from cold and hunger, is more apt to become infected."

Other doctors blamed infection on the atmosphere, a lack of ventilation, or nearby sewer gas. At one Hotel Dieu outbreak, doctors first attributed the problem to infectious air emanating from wounded men on another floor. Hospitals attempted all sorts of ineffective remedies: They repainted rooms, smeared cream of calcium hypochlorite on the walls, baked linens, and filled the wards with smoke.

When a woman giving birth at home became infected, Charles White, the British doctor who blamed women for self-poisoning, suggested that a house's "putrid atmosphere," consisting of a large fire and many people breathing on the mother, could be to blame. His solution: Open the windows. A Rotunda doctor, as well, believed ventilation could prevent infection, and so ordered holes drilled in the hospital's sashes and doors and made sure windows had louvered panes and ceilings had vents. There were twenty-three outbreaks at the Rotunda over the course of a century.

There did not need to be so many women dying, for so long. As early as 1795, Alexander Gordon of Aberdeen, Scotland, had discovered the real cause of the infection—attendants' dirty hands. But physicians were indignant over being blamed, refusing to acknowledge that they could be the source of the scourge. Instead, they kept their "fatal secret," as Gordon called it, and continued carrying the disease.

It was quite a while before anyone else reached that same conclusion. In 1843, Oliver Wendell Holmes of Boston, an anatomy and physiology professor at Harvard, discovered that childbed fever was contagious and that washing hands helped prevent it, although he wasn't sure why. Few, however, wanted to believe his theories, either.

Then, in 1847, Ignaz Semmelweis of Vienna, working in the maternity wards at the Allgemeine Krankenhaus—at one time the world's largest lying-in hospital—discovered microscopic proof of the origins of the disease. "Puerperal fever is caused by conveyance to the pregnant woman of putrid particles derived from living organisms, through the agency of the examining fingers," he declared. "Consequently must I make my confession that God only knows the number of women whom I have consigned prematurely to the grave."

Semmelweis ordered staff hand washing in chlorinated water, and ultimately reduced fever mortality in his hospital from 20 percent to 1 percent. But at the time, he was ridiculed and largely ignored, his own staff sneaking to defy him whenever they could. He died in a state-run insane asylum in 1865.

Not until Pasteur and Lister also determined that hand washing could prevent infection did the practice become routine in hospitals. This led to another medical milestone: the invention of rubber gloves. In 1890, a nurse at Johns Hopkins Hospital developed a rash on her hands from the constant use of disinfectants. The surgeon-in-chief, William Stewart Halsted, asked the Goodyear Rubber Company to design a pair of gloves for her. (The couple later married.) But because those early gloves were awkward to use during obstetrical exams—dulling the sense of touch so that it was difficult to detect cervical dilation or presentation of the fetus—not everyone wore them.

And because not everyone washed effectively, and not everyone wore gloves, childbed fever remained a killer. By the 1920s, the disease accounted for as much as 40 percent of maternal fatalities in American and European hospitals. It wasn't until the 1940s, when antibiotics became widely available, that the malignance of childbed fever became less deadly.

In addition to the high mortality rates, the obstetric practices inside these hospitals were aggressive. One of the more stunning "systems" of delivery was practiced by Dr. William Goodell at Preston Retreat in Philadelphia. There, he administered advance doses of quinine, considered an all-purpose preventive, as well as drugs for constipation, sleeplessness, and headaches. When labor began, nurses would give the woman an enema and a bath; the doctor then ruptured the amniotic sac, applied forceps, and gave the woman ergot when the head appeared, to intensify contractions and reduce blood loss. Finally, he pressed on the abdomen to force out the placenta.

Such systems made maternity hospitals seem more like factories. And with each procedure, doctors, then operating under few regulations or standards, increased the chances of causing more harm. In fact, according to the New York Academy of Medicine's landmark 1933 study called *Maternal Mortality in New York City*, poor hospital care led to the majority of mother and baby deaths. Most of the maternal fatalities were preventable, caused by "ignorance and insufficient training of the attendant." A White House report released shortly thereafter found that mortality was not declining with more hospital births. Equally shocking, infant deaths from birth injuries had jumped nearly 50 percent between 1915 and 1929.

So why were pregnant women—increasingly even middle-class ones—still checking in to hospitals? Because delivering at home, at least in many developed countries, had become impractical. Urban families were crammed into small apartments that left little room for a mother to give birth privately. Fewer midwives were practicing, and doctors were mostly seeing women in hospitals, which—after they instituted hand washing—portrayed themselves as the sterile alternative to a woman's home. Furthermore, women seeking newfangled pain relief options could receive them only in a maternity ward. For a fee.

With more women being shoehorned into hospitals to deliver, the facilities no longer served only charity patients. More and more, they welcomed paying customers. And pay they did. Compared with midwifery services, hospitals were expensive, costing, in the 1920s, half a year's salary.

"The cost was such a burden and a worry that our joy in the child and interest in the birth were under a cloud," one woman said about the high price of hospital care. "Our mothers had their babies delivered for $25 by country doctors, but of course that was before the days of enlightenment. We knew now about prenatal care, anesthesia, and hospitals. The best was none too good, especially when one was in a flutter about something so unusual and dangerous as the birth of a baby."

By 1938 about half of U.S. births were in hospitals. By 1945 the figure had jumped to nearly 80 percent, in part because the federal government was paying for the health care of those married to a serviceman. Also affecting the increase in hospital deliveries was the expansion in private insurance coverage from Blue Cross, which had gone from 4.4 million to 15.7 million policy holders after a national wage freeze forced employers to offer more generous benefits.

By 1955, 99 percent of women were giving birth in hospitals. The same trend was happening elsewhere. In Europe and

Canada, after the Second World War, taxpayer-funded health systems provided medical care to all, regardless of ability to pay. Along with that funding came policies about childbirth and where it should take place: Namely, in a hospital. (This is true even today in America, where health insurers commonly refuse to pay for planned home births, which can cost a mother as much as four thousand dollars, out of pocket, to cover midwifery charges.) In the UK during the 1920s, only about one-fifth of mothers delivered in the hospital. By 1954, the number had reached 64 percent, and by 1991, 99 percent of births took place in hospitals. In Japan, the transition from home to hospital came late, but fast. In 1950, more than 95 percent of women were still giving birth at home. By 1975, only 1.2 percent was. The Netherlands has remained the exception: Nearly 30 percent of births there still take place at home, largely because of an insurance system that offers a financial incentive for them to do so.

HOME AGAIN

Although the class of hospital patients may have changed in the first half of the twentieth century, the culture inside maternity wards did not. Women often were treated shamefully, with little regard to their own wishes—treatment that was all the more stunning to those who may have been the first in their family to deliver in such a place. The hospitals had their protocols, which not even the famous could escape.

When it was time for American anthropologist Margaret Mead to give birth in a New York hospital on the eve of World War II, she tried to import some of what she had learned about how women in Samoa and New Guinea delivered. But she failed. The hospital, after all, had its guidelines, including those that dictated how long she could keep the baby with her and when she could breast-feed. Mead, already a well-known public figure and best-selling author, had asked a young doctor, Benjamin Spock, to be there, to advocate for her to be allowed to breast-feed the baby on demand, rather than the strict every-four-hour feeding schedule that was standard practice then for newborns weighing more than seven pounds. Mead also wanted to keep the child with her in her room overnight, which was forbidden by state law.

"Margaret, of course, wanted breast-feeding. I assume that it was because of all the societies that she'd studied in the South Seas. It was taken for granted that of course a mother breast-feeds. And I think it was my impression that anything that women in the South Seas did was probably right . . . [and] the somewhat *depraved idea,*" Spock said with gravelly emphasis in a documentary years later, "like the one that American women are too tense to be able to breast-feed, she saw that was bogus."

Mead's obstetrician, Claude Heaton, was supposedly interested in indigenous medical practices and told her he would consider her request not to have anesthesia unless it was absolutely necessary. He even showed the nurses a film that Mead had made capturing a postpartum scene in New Guinea and told the staff to cooperate with her wishes.

"And so it came about that at thirty-eight, after many years of experience as a student of child development and of childbirth in remote villages—watching children born on a steep wet hillside, in the 'evil place' reserved for pigs and defecation, or while old women threw stones at the inquisitive children who came to stare at the parturient woman—I was to share in the wartime experience of young wives around the world. My husband had gone away [to England] to take his wartime place, and there was no way of knowing whether I would ever see him again," Mead recalled decades later.

Despite her anthropological credentials, her best-selling books, her amenable doctor, well-briefed nurses, and Spock's attendance, Mead did not have the "natural" birth and unrestricted breast-feeding she had argued for. "They were convinced that as a primipara [woman delivering her first child] I could not be so ready for birth and I was given medication to slow things down," she said. When her daughter finally emerged, she weighed a few ounces over the seven-pound cutoff for more frequent feedings. So the hospital staff made a great concession to let Mead breast-feed the baby more often—every three hours, including at night, rather than every four hours. "According to hospital practice then . . . a baby should go home from the hospital ready to sleep the night through— already, at a few days old, resigned to a world whose imposed rhythms are strange and uncongenial," Mead huffed.

Mead's experience may seem extreme. Yet procedures commonly were worse for the average woman. Hospitals, in an effort to eliminate puerperal infections, had become rigid and methodical. The obstetric ward's obsession with sterility had changed birth entirely. The situation was so grim that in November 1957, a registered nurse wrote to the *Ladies' Home Journal* calling for an investigation into the "tortures that go on in the modern delivery rooms":

> When I first started in my profession, I thought it would be wonderful to help bring new life into this world. I was and am still shocked at the manner in which a mother-to-be is rushed into the delivery room and strapped down with cuffs around her arms and legs and steel clamps over shoulders and chest.
>
> At one hospital I know of it is common practice to take the mother right into the delivery room as soon as she is "prepared." [This preparation would have meant shaved pubic hair and an enema.] Often she is strapped in the lithotomy position, legs in stirrups with knees pulled far apart, for as long as eight hours. On one occasion, an obstetrician informed the nurses on duty that he was going to a dinner and that they should slow up things. The young mother was

taken into the delivery room and strapped down hand and foot with her legs tied together.

I have seen doctors who have charming examination-table manners show traces of sadism in the delivery room. One I know does cutting and suturing operations without anesthetic because he almost lost a patient from an overdose some years ago. He has nurses use a mask to stifle the patient's outcry.

Great strides have been made in maternal care, but some doctors still say, "Tie them down so they won't give us any trouble."

The *Ladies' Home Journal,* filled with Jell-O recipes and ads showing women in aprons standing next to gleaming appliances, tended to put a happy face on all aspects of midcentury domesticity and motherhood. But when the magazine ran that anonymous letter, its readers put down their pots and pans and took up pens to spew their pent-up rage over the indignities of giving birth in a modern American hospital.

Although some hospitals had already begun to "allow" natural childbirth and lying-in—where the baby and mother could stay together—many women were still experiencing some of what the nurse had written about to the magazine. Half of the respondents to her letter said that they had endured the ordeal of having their babies held back from being born because the doctor was not available. Others recounted how they had their wrists, legs, or shoulders strapped to the table or stirrups because the hospital was worried about a mother contaminating the "sterile field" they had worked so hard to achieve.

A woman from New York had leather cuffs placed on her wrists and legs while she was left alone for nearly eight hours until the actual delivery. A mother from Montana said six months after she delivered, her legs were just beginning to feel normal because they had been held in stirrups for so long. Nurses wrote in to defend the practices. One, from Rhode Island, said, "Lay people do not understand why hands are tied. They are cuffed comfortably at the patient's sides to prevent contamination. . . . Is it so difficult to understand why her legs are in padded stirrups? From waist to toes she is covered with sterile drapes. The doctor uses sterile gloves and a sterile gown. Infection was the greatest cause of death not too many years ago, so with the elimination of contamination mother and child are healthy and alive!"

Another nurse, from California, wondered what the fuss was about, saying stirrups were "quite comfortable during labor." And a third, from Texas, explained that shoulder clamps were for the mother's own protection. "They keep her from falling off the table in case of emergency—if her head has to be lowered quickly, as in shock," she said.

It's no wonder that women, fighting to break free of real and metaphorical shackles in the 1960s and '70s, sought alternative places to give birth. And the most radical among them would insist on a very old option: delivering at home, surrounded now by ferns, shag rugs, and psychedelic posters. This latest round of home births—intentional and mostly among the middle class—peaked at around 5 percent of all deliveries in places such as California in the late 1970s.

But the trend wasn't only evident on the West Coast. When Noreen Mattis was a nursing student in Rhode Island in the 1960s, she never saw a conscious woman give birth. It wasn't until after she had her first daughter in a Catholic hospital in the late 1960s —she labored alone, was given a pill that knocked her out just before the baby emerged, and tore badly—that she realized how awful the situation was. Her own experience propelled her to become a childbirth educator, telling a woman what to expect, how to handle contractions and pain. It was a small way for her to help change the system, one group of mothers at a time. Sometimes, at the end of class, a woman would approach her and ask if she would help her give birth at home. Mattis often consented, understanding all too well how many pregnant women felt at the time.

"It was like a religious fervor," she said. Mattis would get a call in the middle of the night, meet a midwife and a liberal obstetrician at the house, and cheerfully help bring a new life into the world. Mostly, she kept these home births a secret. "You were very careful who you ever told," said Mattis, who today works as an administrator at a Providence maternity hospital.

Would she ever attend or encourage a home birth now? Absolutely not, Mattis said, because hospitals have evolved to become, well, more hospitable to laboring women.

There is, however, one distinct group of American women still giving birth at home: the devoutly religious. Many of them refuse to enroll with health insurers that cover abortions; they are modest about exposing themselves to men; and they want to keep birth within the family and out of institutional control.

Although doctors have always advised against home births— a former president of the American College of Obstetrics and Gynecology said, "Home birth is child abuse in its earliest form"—many have been equally opposed to what was supposed to be the happy medium: birth centers.

BIRTH CENTERS

The first model birth center was opened in 1975 by Ruth Lubic in an Upper East Side town house in New York. The hippie era of home deliveries had scared a lot of birth professionals. First, because there was not always someone present who was licensed to catch the baby, and second, the mother's political views against a hospital may have been so strident that she would have refused to go to the emergency room if something went wrong. There had to be a middle ground, they believed, between the lack of a safety net at home and the dehumanizing hospital.

Lubic was the director of the Maternity Center Association, which had existed since the 1930s promoting more natural childbirth. "We have tried to establish an alternative for these women— a setting as much like a home as possible but where a medical emergency can be handled," Lubic said when the facility first opened. "If necessary, we could get mother, baby or both to our backup hospital—Lenox Hill—within 11 minutes."

The association's state-licensed facility, called The Childbearing Center, was staffed by nurse-midwives and obstetricians who allowed women to give birth in any safe position they wanted. They could also hold and keep their babies immediately after birth. The waiting room, the home's original foyer, had an oriental carpet, historic sculptures of fetal development, and a wrought-iron staircase with a wooden railing. If that wasn't enough enticement over a hospital setting, the lower level, designed for women in labor, had a small sitting room and garden where staff encouraged walking and waiting. One delivery room was decorated in bright orange, another in blue. Both had leatherette reclining chairs, hospital beds, baby scales, bassinettes, flowery curtains, and plants.

The Childbearing Center was defined almost as much by what it did not have or do. There were no stirrups, no general anesthesia, and therefore no ability to perform C-sections. They did not do routine enemas, pubic hair shaving, or episiotomies. And women could leave within twelve hours of bearing the baby. The total charge, including prenatal care, childbirth classes, and postpartum care, was $550 in 1975, about half of what doctor visits and a hospital delivery would have cost. In fact, many early birth centers became magnets for the uninsured, who could not afford hospitals.

As more and more birth centers opened, the American Academy of Pediatrics and the American College of Obstetricians and Gynecologists became alarmed, saying no one knew whether they were safe. In 1989, the *New England Journal of Medicine* published a landmark survey that followed 11,814 low-risk women admitted for labor and delivery to eighty-four freestanding birth centers in the United States. Doctors tracked them and their infants through delivery or transfer to a hospital and for at least four weeks after birth. The results were very similar to those in hospitals. The report concluded that birth centers were a safe and acceptable alternative to the hospital for low-risk women, especially those who had had children before.

Suddenly, it seemed, hospitals had competition.

Unwilling to cede any business to birth centers, hospitals got busy co-opting their warm and fuzzy features. Some created their own birthing rooms or suites amid the usual maternity services. By the late 1970s there were more than one thousand of these rooms, decorated with plants and equipped with seven-thousand-dollar motorized "borning" beds—adjustable contraptions designed to look like traditional furniture. Some hospital rooms had nightstands that transformed into baby monitors and bureaus that folded out to become instrument holders. Other institutions went even further, offering post-delivery candlelight celebration dinners. But still, this was mostly standard maternity care in disguise.

There were hospitals that took a more purist approach, opening birth centers on or near their grounds. That's what happened in 1997 when Cambridge Hospital in Massachusetts opened the Cambridge Birth Center across the street, in what was formerly a single-family Victorian house. The first year, when the staff scraped together money to advertise in the phone book, the Cambridge Birth Center had just 7 deliveries; in 2005 it had 103, Alejandra Torres's natural labor and delivery among them.

When she and her husband, Elias, arrived at the Cambridge Birth Center in 2003 to have their first child, the idea of birth outside a hospital seemed extreme to Alejandra's mother, who, two thousand miles away in Florida, continued to implore the couple via telephone to go to the hospital.

"I'm looking at the hospital out the window!" Elias told her. Indeed, the hospital was so close one could walk—or roll on a gurney—across the street in case of emergency transfer. But that street is more like a line in the sand, separating totally natural births from those laden with monitors and surgical equipment.

At the birth center, guests are on a first-name basis with the staff; the receptionist often answers the phone while holding someone's baby; a plaster cast of a pregnant belly hangs on the wall; and the kitchen, with its oatmeal and coffee, is available to all. New parents share a queen-size mahogany Ethan Allen bed. There is no pain medicine but plenty of food, drink, psychological support, massage, and time in the tub. All the comforts of home, with an infant resuscitation table waiting in the hall, out of sight, just in case. Because their first experience there was so pleasant, the Torreses returned to the birth center in 2005 to have their second baby. Offered the room of their choice, they settled in the one with the largest tub, and Alejandra gave birth on a simple stool.

Despite such personalized services and happy customers, the number of birth centers has dwindled. For one thing, epidurals are not available at birth centers. Also, high-risk pregnancies—which include everything from women over 35 to those weighing more than 250 pounds to those with previous C-sections—are barred from birth centers because of malpractice insurance policies. Furthermore, birth centers are facing worsening financial conditions. Independent birth centers—those that are not affiliated with a hospital—must bear the intense cost of skyrocketing malpractice insurance. Centers that have been open for two decades without a single malpractice suit have still seen their insurance rates jump 200 percent in a single year, with more increases likely. (Rates vary depending on how litigious the state is.) Couple that crippling economic fact with decreasing reimbursements from health maintenance organizations and few can continue practicing. Some birth centers have been forced to affiliate with a deep-pocketed hospital, seeking shelter under its insurance umbrella, but that has not always worked out. Take, for example, Lubic's pioneering birth center in New York City. The facility, renamed the Elizabeth Seton Childbearing Center, moved downtown to affiliate with St. Vincent's Hospital, but the hospital closed the facility in 2003 because the midwives' malpractice insurance premiums had become too expensive. It was the industry's most high-profile closure so far.

WHERE WE GIVE BIRTH TODAY

Those shut out of birth centers are now reverting to the home or the hospital. In the late 1990s, Pamela Udy had two cesareans, both of which she believed were unnecessary. When it was time to deliver again, in 2001, the thirty-year-old Mormon mom in Ogden, Utah, did not want to go through another operation with a long recovery period. But hospital obstetricians were balking about allowing her to have a vaginal birth after a cesarean (called a VBAC, pronounced veeback).

So Udy convinced her husband that delivering in their ranch home would be a good idea. (The practice of having a VBAC at home is now becoming prevalent enough that "home birth after cesarean" has its own acronym: HBAC.) Udy found an experienced midwife, had an ultrasound to make sure the baby and placenta were in safe positions, and tried to keep the plan a secret from her mother, who would surely disapprove. "I was not following doctors' orders," Udy admitted.

When labor began on a Monday morning in October 2001,

she sent her two boys to school and did what someone in her position during the colonial era would have done. She called her women together. The group consisted of a midwife and a pair of doulas. They watched a video and blew up some pink and red balloons with a helium tank. Udy walked around the house, leaned against the couch when a contraction warranted, labored on the toilet for a while, and then delivered her daughter in bed.

While she took a bath, the midwife and doulas cleaned the bedroom and bought her a special takeout sandwich she was craving. Udy was sitting on the couch holding her newborn when her sons came home from school and said, "Hey, Mom, here's the work we did today."

"That's great," she said. "Here's what I did today!"

Despite Udy's success story, doctors do consider VBACs at home to be risky. But what about low-risk births? Are home deliveries safe for the average woman today? A 1992 study looked at seventeen hundred women attended by midwives between 1971 and 1989 at The Farm, a commune–cum–birth center in Tennessee. Researchers compared those home-style births with fourteen thousand doctor-assisted ones in hospitals during the same time. The home births were found to be—like birth center deliveries— "as safe as" the hospital ones.

European research has reached similar conclusions. In 1997, the University of Copenhagen looked at the outcomes of twenty-four thousand births. In that study, those who delivered at home actually fared better; infants were in better condition, and the mothers had fewer lacerations, a lower rate of induction, and fewer interventions, including the use of forceps, than those in the hospital. There were no maternal deaths. A 1996 Dutch study of two thousand births also showed that birthing at home was safer than the hospital, especially for women having their second or third babies.

Regardless, 98 percent of North American and British

women today choose to deliver in a hospital. Despite all the evidence to the contrary, women still believe hospitals are the safest—or the only—choice. Thankfully, hospitals have updated their appearance and attitude. Shackles, stirrups, and knock-'em-out drugs are gone. Women labor and deliver in the same room—decorated perhaps with mauve wallpaper and pretty beach scenes—equipped with a private shower and a nurse who may be willing to look at a birth plan.

There have been other, more subtle, changes, as well.

When Carolyn Digiammo went into labor in 2005, she and her husband, Joseph, left their suburban house and headed for Brigham and Women's Hospital, formerly the Boston Lying-In, where Bridget Logan died of childbed fever a little more than one hundred years before. The Digiammos pulled up to the main entrance at 1:00 a.m., handed the car keys to a valet parking attendant, and took the elevator to what is now called the Center for Labor and Birth. Years ago, the floor was known as Labor and Delivery, but at some point, the latter word was no longer considered politically correct. (I have used *delivery* in various forms throughout the book because I believe the word no longer implies that someone besides the mother is taking credit for the birth; a mother can deliver herself of a child.)

Once admitted, the Digiammos settled into a private room with a rocker, a television, a chair that converts to a sleeper, and a bathroom with a shower stall. The privacy is a luxury in contrast to the shared rooms and group showers hospitals had just thirty years ago. Once the staff hooked her up to an epidural, IV bag, and fetal monitor, Carolyn was happily comfortable. The room was dimmed and quiet except for the constant sound of baby James's heartbeat pounding over a speaker and the nurse shuffling through printouts of contractions and vital signs. Carolyn rested, while her husband, on the recliner, fielded the occasional cell phone call. With the staff out of the room, she relaxed, feeling no pain as her cervix dilated. The nurse returned, checked her progress, and asked if she was ready to start pushing.

At 8:23 a.m., Carolyn called *her* women together. Or, more precisely, the nurse did. In an instant, three more women appeared: There was the attending obstetrician overseeing things from the foot of the bed, a medical student hoping to catch the baby, and an outspoken resident—quick with wisecracks about male obstetricians—manually stretching the perineum. The machines buzzed, everyone donned her rubber gloves. A nurse placed a splash mat beneath Carolyn and a clip on her toe to measure the oxygen in her blood.

At 8:46 a.m., James Digiammo was born. Cheers erupted in the room. The nurse put a secure identity band on the boy's ankle, gave him a few drops of sugar water on his tongue—a new procedure for infant comfort—injected him in the thigh with a standard shot of vitamin K, which a doctor first discovered in 1937 could help prevent a potentially fatal bleeding disorder in newborns, and wrapped him in a blanket. He never squawked. She then offered Carolyn apple juice in a paper cup and within two hours transferred them via gurney to a private room on a postpartum floor with a magnificent view of the city.

By lunchtime a cleaning crew had descended on the birthing room and by 2:00 p.m. a seventeen-year-old was moaning in the same spot, with the same nurse, having the very same sort of epidural wired to her back, just inches above her tattoo. Unlike Bridget Logan's time 125 years ago, there was no longer any stigma associated with this single teenager being there.

Deliveries at home and in birth centers have been statistically proven to be as safe as those in hospitals, where, not incidentally, one's chances of having a cesarean soar just because you walk through the door. But despite all the apparent options for Westernized expectant mothers, we have almost as little choice in where we will deliver as the Mbuti pygmy does, due to limited insurance coverage, cultural norms, and the deep fear many women have about how dangerous birth can be. There are, and always have been, trade-offs in decisions about where a child should be born, especially in terms of comfort, support, and intervention. Weighing those options, women still want to give birth where they feel most safe. And for all but a fraction of those pregnant today, that place is on a bed that can—if necessary—be wheeled into the operating room, surrounded by machines, and attached to electrodes and a catheter that drips anesthetic directly to the spine.

4 PAIN RELIEF

PREGNANT WOMEN HAVE always dreaded the pain of childbirth and have done just about anything to avoid feeling it. Five thousand years ago, the Egyptians and Indians made use of opium, from which we would later derive morphine. The Greeks chewed willow bark, the predecessor to aspirin. The people of the Andes had their coca leaves, the basis for cocaine. And myrrh might not have been just for the baby Jesus. Some people believe that the Wise Men brought that gift as much to help Mary ease her pain of labor. Women have drunk wine and poppy juice, eaten mandrake and hemp. They've been hypnotized and lulled by the power of positive suggestion. They've been offered Demerol, Nubain, and Stadol, and even had ether and olive oil injected into the rectum, a method that women in the early twentieth century found effective when combined with a small dose of a barbiturate.

Drugs aside, many in myth and reality have sworn they would give up anything to avoid the agony of childbirth. Even sex. The Greek goddess Artemis was so terrified by her mother's suffering at her own birth that she asked Zeus for the favor of eternal virginity. She changed her mind, though, seduced Endymion, and ended up giving birth to fifty daughters.

Mere mortals, also unable to resist the lures of sex, have sung, chanted, prayed, swayed, and walked to reduce pain. They've eaten cassowary anus and swamp eel, hoping to make the birth canal slippery. Women have bathed in cold water during pregnancy as a pain preventive. They have tried acupuncture, aromatherapy, hypnosis, biofeedback, massage, water injections, and hot baths. Some cultures believed that evil spirits were the source of the woman's pain and turned their attention to fighting the invisible demons, rather than attending to the mother-to-be. Other indigenous peoples, from Siberia to the Sudan, would demand confessions from the woman in labor. Did she commit adultery? If she did not answer truthfully, they believed, her birth would be extremely painful.

In 1841, Mr. Rowbotham, a London chemist, published a pamphlet outlining a new "fruit diet," which he said would help a woman avoid pain in birth. His wife had suffered greatly with her first two deliveries, and so a couple of months before she was due to have her third child, he prescribed her to eat foods "free of earthy and bony matter."

Mr. Rowbotham had read that an embryo is mostly fluid, a gelatinous pulp that gradually hardens a skeletal core. And so he had this thought: If the fetus slowly consolidates in firmness, drawing its bony particles from its mother's blood, what if you changed the mother's blood composition by restricting her diet of foods believed to harden bones? If the baby wasn't bony, he reasoned, the fetus could slip through the birth canal without causing pain.

The diet called for eating lots of ripe, acidic fruits, eschewing bread and pastry. For breakfast, his wife would eat an apple and an orange, lemon juice with sugar, two or three roasted apples, sometimes boiled whole with potatoes. In the afternoon she'd get an orange, an apple, or some grapes followed by more lemon juice. Dinner would be more apples and oranges, rice boiled in milk, with the occasional figs and raisins stewed in it. The chemist said her swollen limbs subsided, and she became so light and active she could run up and down the stairs. The midwife reported, "A more easy labor I never witnessed—I never saw such a thing and I have been at a great many labors in my time! The child, a boy, was finely proportioned and exceedingly soft, his bones resembling gristle." The woman was allowed to eat "bony" foods postpartum to help the baby grow via her breast milk.

The fruit diet may sound silly, but for centuries folk and quackish pain remedies were all a laboring woman had. *The Byrth of Mankynde* instructed sixteenth-century midwives to comfort women with the simple means available then, offering "meate and drinke"; baths; suppositories; anointments, including the grease of hens, ducks, and geese; olive oil; linseed oil; fenugreek oil or white lily oil; and kind words, "giving her good hope of a speedful deliverance, encouraging . . . her to patience and tolerance, bidding her to hold in her breath as much as she may, also striking gently with her hands her belly about the navel, for that helpeth to dispel the birth downward."

Doctors, on the other hand, were more focused on trying to eradicate pain. One famous American obstetrician, Joseph B. DeLee, believed that pain was dangerous to anyone who experienced it. In 1920, DeLee, who practiced in Chicago, said that giving birth felt like falling on a pitchfork; and birth for the baby was so painful and harmful that delivery was akin to its head being crushed in a door. In an effort to reduce trauma and pain for mother and child, DeLee devised the "prophylactic forceps operation," which simply involved giving the mother a large episiotomy, or cut to widen the mouth of the birth canal, inserting the equipment, and pulling out the baby. The procedure popularized forceps use in the United States for decades and likely caused more pain and trauma to mother and child than anything else.

Today, doctors believe birth is not normally painful for the child. However, studies have shown that labor can cause the most severe pain a woman will feel. Its intensity is almost always greatest among first-time mothers, younger women, those with bigger babies, those with a history of menstrual problems, and those who were unprepared for what to expect. A natural birth without the pain is possible but rare—only about 2 or 3 percent of women report having one.

WHY IT HURTS

The uterus, when not home to a fetus, is the size of a fist and weighs less than two ounces. At term, that organ is the largest and strongest muscle in the body, weighing as much as two pounds, baby and placenta excluded. It is a smooth muscle and works on autopilot, just like the heart. In a peak of contraction, it feels as if a mechanical crank is tightening a tourniquet around the abdomen, a sensation so severe that those experiencing it find it impossible to talk, think about other things, or even keep their eyes open. Contractions are like a rhythmic, intense charley horse. This tightening, at its fiercest lasting about thirty seconds, stimulates nerve fibers that record pain. The stronger the contraction the more forcefully the long muscles that run the length of the uterus pull up on the circular muscles that control the opening of the cervix, and the more it hurts. When the uterus is contracting, blood flow to it is restricted and waste products build up, which causes a burning sensation. (Contractions, and the pain, continue after birth to bring the uterus back to its old shape.)

There is also pain associated with the opening of the cervix. Pelvic ligaments and joints are stretched the way a circus clown might prepare a long balloon before twisting it into a purple dachshund. The pressure from the moving baby can pull on the fallopian tubes and ovaries. The head compresses the bowels and the bladder. If the baby is not in the perfect position to come out, its head and spine may scrape and press against the woman's back and other soft tissues for hours without relief. At the point when the baby is about to thrust through the exit, the stretching can become so intense that the sensation is sometimes called the ring of fire. (To sample this feeling, take your index fingers and hook them at the corners of your mouth. Now pull. Pull some more. Keep pulling until you see stars. You get the idea.)

Forceps stretch the vaginal opening wider than it might naturally extend (continue pulling at the corners of your mouth until your lips crack and bleed), and they can pull down a baby before everything has opened (quickly tug once on the corners of your mouth as hard as you can). In botched cases, forceps have shredded a mother's soft tissues and injured babies by ripping off an ear, breaking a nose, denting a skull. Today, forceps and the vacuum extractor—a small cup attached by suction to the fetal skull to help the doctor pull out the child—are most often used when the mother has an epidural or some other pain medication and is too numb to effectively push.

There's another source of pain that has been harder to medicate: Indignities. How much does it hurt to have an unwanted procedure such as an enema? To have your pubic hair shaved? To be strapped down on a delivery table? To have your legs in stirrups for hours? To be roughed up by the hospital staff, as one woman claimed in a letter to the *Ladies' Home Journal*?

"The anesthetist hit me, pushed my head back, sticking her fingers into my throat so that I couldn't breathe," a woman from Homewood, Illinois, complained in a letter to the magazine in 1958. "She kept saying 'You're killing your baby. Do you want a misfit or a dead baby? You're killing it every time you yell for the doctor.' When my husband saw my bruised neck, face and arms, he questioned the doctor and was told that first mothers knock themselves around."

Was birth always painful? Probably not. The evolutionary consequence of humans having developed their neocortex, or thinking brain, is that we are more sensitive to discomfort as well as pleasure than our earliest ancestors may have been. Modern life has given us other problems—from rickets to big-headed babies—that could contribute to how much it hurts to give birth. Even the Western use of chairs, any yoga instructor will say, can cause a tight pelvis, as opposed to the more open pelvises seen among people who squat during daily activities.

Some cultural and religious inhibitions have also contributed to birth pain. Samoan tradition forbids women to express pain. The Scientologist religion decrees that women should not make any noise during labor, nor should anyone else in the room, mostly for the benefit of the emerging child. "If you're quiet, you help reduce the amount of negative effect it could have on him in the future," says a church spokesman. "You would want the mother to be as quiet as possible because if the mother is screaming, 'Oh, my god, this is the most painful thing in my life!' . . . this could have a negative effect on the child." Quiet has also been the norm in the labor wards of Tokyo and in the rural villages of Benin, where the silent, stoic endurance of labor pain is a Bariba woman's principal avenue to social prestige. But it's no small feat being quiet. Yelling and grunting are ways of gaining energy, managing exertion, and dealing with the pain. Think of an army storming a hill without shouting a battle cry, or someone trained in the martial arts silently attacking a pile of cinder blocks. It is certainly unnatural, to be hushed when such work is required.

At other times, cultural taboos, especially among the Victorians, restricted women from assuming unflattering positions, encouraging them instead to deliver lying down, a pose that may look ladylike but does not work very well for the mechanics of labor and can be excruciating if the woman is in back labor, when the baby's head is pressing against her spine. Of course, most women who labor in bed today are hooked up to epidurals, something Victorian culture would have relished; instead, Victorian women bowed to society's dictates that they be passive victims. "Neither appreciation of, nor desire for physical excellence sufficiently exists among refined women of our day," one American doctor said in the 1880s. "Our young women are too willing to be delicate, fragile, and incapable of endurance."

The women of the Victorian era didn't just act frail. They were frail. Because it was fashionable for the upper classes to have large families, pregnancies were stacked one after another, aided by the fact that the rich rarely breast fed, causing the resumption of ovulation sooner after a birth. Successive pregnancies, combined with poor eating habits and little exercise, left these women haggard. On top of that, wearing whale-bone corsets constricted the abdomen, and often caused digestive troubles, miscarriage, or a displaced womb.

Birth hurts because women don't have roomy pelvises. It hurts because women expect it to. And it hurts because women have been physically and emotionally restricted by societal norms and conventions from doing what might make them feel better, whether it's shouting, squatting, or having company there to support them.

The only thing as consistent as birth pain has been the search to eradicate it, pharmaceutically.

GIVE ME DRUGS

When he was just starting out as a doctor in the early 1800s, James Young Simpson of Edinburgh watched as a woman writhing in agony had a cancerous breast amputated. The sight was so dreadful that he considered quitting medicine. Instead, he turned his attention to finding a cure for pain. He believed he had found that cure on January 19, 1847, when he became the first to use diethyl ether during labor, on a woman with a pelvis deformed by rickets. She periodically inhaled the strong fumes of the clear liquid, becoming either groggy or unconscious, depending on how much she took each time.

A thirteenth-century Spanish alchemist had discovered ether, and in the centuries that followed, it was used to relieve pain. By the 1820s college students were taking the drug for fun, holding "ether frolics." When Simpson tried ether he found it to be an effective anesthetic, but he did not like its odor, felt the large quantities necessary to keep the woman relieved over hours of labor impractical, and was displeased by the lung irritation it caused. (He did not then know that ether could be toxic to the liver and kidneys.)

So Simpson began to look for an alternative. Sitting at the head of his dining table, he tested all sorts of drugs on himself. One day an assistant recommended they try chloroform, a relatively new discovery. They obtained a sample, filled tumblers with the "curious liquid," and drank it straight. At once, they became very chatty. Then incoherent. Then they crashed to the floor. When Simpson came to, he knew he was on to something. They continued to experiment with chloroform, albeit more gingerly, and even persuaded some women to join in the tests, including Simpson's niece, Miss Petrie, who cried out under its influence, "I'm an angel! Oh, I'm an angel!"

Simpson administered chloroform for the first time in a maternity case, to the wife of a doctor, in her second pregnancy. After her cervix was fully dilated, he took a half teaspoonful of chloroform, moistened his pocket handkerchief with it, rolled the handkerchief into the shape of a funnel, and placed the opening over her mouth and nostrils. He repeated this every ten minutes as the agent evaporated. The child was born within twenty-five minutes, as the mother lay sound asleep. When she awoke, she was astonished that labor was over and the child was hers. She was so delighted that she gave her baby girl the middle name Anaesthesia.

Though Simpson's accomplishment was heralded by women, it was not celebrated by all. According to some biblical interpretations, women must suffer during birth—it's Eve's curse. In Genesis 3:16, God says to Eve, "I will greatly multiply thy sorrow and thy conception; in sorrow thou shalt bring forth children." For centuries, those words were the single greatest obstacle for women to receive pain relief while giving birth. Some were even burned at the stake for trying to find ways to ease their suffering. In 1591, a woman named Eufame Macalyane of Edinburgh asked a midwife to place a special stone under her head and give her a potion—said to have included the finger, toe, and knee joints of dug-up corpses—to erase labor pain. King James VI ordered her burned alive for attempting such a heretical thing as trying to ease her birth pain. The midwife also was executed, for witchcraft.

The Scottish Church was no less outraged over Simpson's use of chloroform. But Simpson was not about to wither before the pulpit. Armed with his own biblical passages committed to memory, he recited a quote from Genesis 2: 21–22 to prove his point that God did not condone suffering. The verses say, "And the Lord God *caused a deep sleep* to fall upon Adam, and he slept: and he took one of his ribs, and closed up the flesh instead thereof; And the rib, which the Lord God had taken from man, made he a woman, and brought her unto the man" (emphasis added). Simpson read those words to say that God did not want suffering to be the by-product of creating another, which is why He essentially anesthetized Adam. Simpson also argued that the word *sorrow,* from Genesis 3:16, had another meaning in Hebrew: "to work." The Bible could be saying that women had to work hard during childbirth but did not necessarily have to feel pain. Simpson even published a pamphlet called the *Answer to the Religious Objections Advanced Against the Employment of Anaesthetic Agents in Midwifery and Surgery*. In it he quoted James 4:17, which says that if one is capable of doing something good and does not do it—that is a sin.

But clerics would not be swayed. They argued that chloroform was a decoy of Satan and criticized Simpson's interpretation of Eve being born of Adam's rib by saying there was no pain or suffering in the Garden of Eden. The biblical Paradise was a state of Innocence. Until Eve sinned.

Meanwhile, in mid-nineteenth-century America, a young Boston doctor named Walter Channing, grandson of a signer of the Declaration of Independence, was considering using ether in his obstetrical practice. Channing was a brilliant and spirited man. After graduating from Harvard he had studied in London and Edinburgh and became Harvard Medical School's first professor of midwifery. He was also the first to diagnose anemia in pregnancy, and he learned how to do blood transfusions on pregnant women. But his best-known contribution is for his involvement in the first documented case of using ether anesthesia for birth in America, on May 7, 1847, about four months after Simpson had tried it across the Atlantic.

Channing, familiar with the enduring religious controversy over pain relief, sought advice from the more liberal Unitarian Church, which his brother had helped found. The church's response was that human ingenuity, if used to relieve pain, was a God-given power. Though the religion question seemed settled, at least in his mind, Channing faced other unexpected criticism, from a fellow doctor, the reactionary Charles Delucena Meigs of Philadelphia. Meigs believed that every twinge and agony associated with birth helped inspire the mother to love her baby more. Birth pain was an unavoidable fact of life, Meigs said, and anesthesia was not worth the risk to mother or doctor. "What sufficient motive have I to risk the death of one in a thousand in a questionable attempt to abrogate one of the general conditions of man?" Meigs wrote.

Channing's reply to Meigs did not address anesthesia's safety, which had not yet been extensively studied, in part because doctors had no way to measure the strength of contractions and knew little about fetal circulatory and metabolic functions. Instead, Channing focused his argument on how pain did not have to be, and had not always been, a given in birth, citing various indigenous cultures that seemed to have an easier time delivering a child. He sarcastically concluded, "By some divines, these symptoms, and particularly pain, have been considered as a standing and unchangeable punishment of the original disobedience of woman . . .

86

[but] I was induced to believe pain does not accompany child-bearing by an immutable decree of Heaven."

Channing's first ether case was an emergency. He was called to the home of a twenty-three-year-old woman, anonymous except for the No. 124 he used to document her story. She had been in labor for two days. The fetus had descended into the pelvis and had been there for some time. A doctor already on the scene had given her an opiate—probably morphine, which was then known as laudanum—and a little belladonna ointment on the cervix to dilate it, without any luck. When Channing arrived, he saw that her vagina was swollen and hot; the child's scalp was also swollen "and protruded as a tumor of conical shape through the firm ring formed by the undilated and undilatable os uteri," meaning the cervix. Channing knew he had to act fast, and he broke out his forceps. He also sent the doctor out to get ether as he began to pull with the iron hands.

"The application was perfectly easy and I made an extracting effort, which was attended with very severe pain," Channing recalled. The doctor returned. Channing instructed him to hold an ether-saturated sponge to the woman's mouth and nose. The patient refused it at first. But she finally consented, breathed it in, coughed slightly, and within a minute was unconscious. Her body jerked, as if she was falling asleep. They asked her her name. She did not respond. So Channing tugged on the forceps again. A contraction aided their efforts. The head advanced. Birth seemed to be imminent.

"But at length the head again became firmly fixed, and this to a degree that prevented its being moved by any such force as I believed it safe to employ," Channing explained. He removed the forceps, and the effects of the ether wore off. She screamed for more pain relief. "Put it to my mouth—I shall faint—you must!'" There was no more ether. They had to send for more. Meanwhile, the situation was quickly deteriorating. Channing reached for a destructive tool. He perforated the baby's cranium, fixed a hook, and pulled. The woman, already in great pain, screamed in agony and thought the baby was out. But the craniotomy was not complete. Finally, more ether arrived. They put the sponge to her face. She saw spots. Her ears rang, and then she blacked out. Channing tugged again on the head, and after much effort the mutilated child was born—killed by the extraction efforts. The woman's recovery—at least the physical part—would be fine, Channing reported.

For all the drama involved in Channing's initial use of ether, he did not know that there had been another case, far more successful, about a month earlier in Boston. Henry Wadsworth Longfellow's second wife, Fanny, asked dentist Nathan Cooley Keep to administer ether for the birth of her third child, a girl. Mother and baby were healthy.

"I never was better or got through a confinement so comfortably," Fanny Longfellow wrote to her sister-in-law. "Two other ladies I know have since followed my example successfully, and I feel proud to be the pioneer to less suffering for poor, weak womankind. This is certainly the greatest blessing of this age."

Despite the eventual notoriety of these early cases, the use of ether and chloroform did not become widespread quickly. Religious and moral issues aside, such pain relief was still an inexact science. More than a year after his first attempt with chloroform, Simpson was still using only a silk handkerchief, sprinkled with an unmeasured amount of the liquid, to smother the patient. How much to administer was more artful than precise. "Generally, I believe, we pour two or three drachms on the handkerchief at once, and more in a minute, if no sufficient effect is produced, and we stop when sonorous respiration begins," Simpson said. Such imprecision scared many doctors from trying it.

In an effort to impose some standards on how to administer the agent, the American Medical Association Committee on Obstetrics recommended in 1848 that doctors pour one-eighth of an ounce of chloroform onto a folded handkerchief, which the mother should breathe in with each contraction. Although doctors later developed rubber masks attached to canisters, those gadgets were not widely available, and doctors often used what was on hand, from woolen gloves to nightcaps.

"If there is no one present to assist me in the final stages of labor, I have the expectant mother hold a drinking glass with the bottom filled with cotton and upon which the chloroform is poured, then have them hold the glass over their nose. When their hands become unsteady and the glass falls away from the nose, I know they are sufficiently asleep to give them relief and I continue to accelerate the delivery," said one physician of the time.

Despite the relief chloroform and ether provided, there were drawbacks to the drugs. For one thing, the woman could inhale anesthesia only just before the baby came out because taking it sooner could ease the contractions and stall the birth. There also were dangerous side effects, including maternal hemorrhage and breathing difficulties for the newborn. Channing believed that ether did not cross the placenta and therefore did not affect the baby. To prove his theory, he sniffed the end of a cut umbilical cord. But if he had smelled the newborn's breath, as others did, he would have detected the lingering presence of the pungent drug. It was not until 1877, some thirty years after those earliest obstetric anesthesia cases, that a Swiss doctor had proof—and the public finally accepted—the fact that the drug passes through the placenta and into the child's system.

Surprisingly, the greatest obstacle separating anesthesia from the general public had nothing to do with safety. The debate remained fixed on religion and morality. That finally changed when Queen Victoria, head of the Church of England, inhaled chloroform during her delivery of Prince Leopold in April of 1853. After the birth, her general physician, Sir James Clark, sent a cable to Simpson, who had encouraged the queen to try chloroform for the birth of the prince, her eighth child. "The Queen had chloroform exhibited to her during her late confinement. . . . It was not at any time given so strongly as to render the Queen insensible, and an ounce of chloroform was scarcely consumed during the whole time," Clark reported to Simpson. "Her Majesty was greatly pleased with the effect, and she certainly never has had a better recovery."

Simpson was elated. He had hoped the queen's endorsement would silence his critics and make anesthesia accepted worldwide. His wish came true. Women on both sides of the Atlantic finally embraced what became fashionably known as chloroform *à la reine.* John Snow, the doctor whose specific duty it was to administer chloroform to the queen, became a sought-after commodity. One mother-to-be, while Snow was giving her chloroform, said she would not inhale any more of it unless he told her word for word what the queen had said when she was taking it. "Her Majesty," Dr. Snow replied, "asked no questions until she had breathed very much longer than you have; and if you will only go on in loyal imitation, I will tell you everything." By the time the woman woke up, Snow had departed.

Although the English medical journal *Lancet* wrote a scathing editorial criticizing Snow for potentially putting the queen's life at risk by using anesthesia, there was no widespread outrage. And four years later, when Victoria used chloroform for the birth of Princess Beatrice, there was no public condemnation at all. Most people by then had overcome their moral and religious objections.

However, the use of anesthesia was limited to a small number of pregnant women, primarily the upper class, who could afford drug-toting physicians over empty-handed midwives. Indeed, society women would continue to search for even more ways to eliminate the agony of birth. By 1914, a new and wondrous technique had caught the attention of these matrons: Twilight Sleep.

TWILIGHT SLEEP

Five years before American women won the right to vote, the burgeoning feminist movement sought to banish the suffering of childbirth once and for all. The activists heard about a new childbirth method at the Frauenklinik in Freiburg, Germany, where doctors had discovered that by combining the amnesiac scopolamine—later called "scope" or "the bomb"—with morphine, a woman in labor could be made to fall into a semiconscious state and emerge hours later with a baby in her arms, remembering nothing that happened in between. In truth, she'd feel pain; she just would not remember it.

Upper-class pregnant women descended upon the facility, located on the edge of the Black Forest, to partake in *Dämmerschlaf,* or Twilight Sleep. There, they would stay in blue tinted rooms, furnished with a little crib, a big white leather recliner, a lounge, and a table. The door was padded. The floors were concrete.

When contractions became less than four minutes apart, the mother would ring a bell, and the doctors would arrive with the injection; the room was deliberately kept dark and quiet to help her fall into a finely balanced clouded consciousness. About thirty minutes after the first shot, the staff would show her an object, and another thirty minutes later they would ask whether she remembered what she saw. If she did, she'd get another injection. Once she was under the spell of Twilight Sleep, the doctor would bandage her eyes with gauze and stuff oil-soaked wads of cotton in her ears, so her own screaming would not wake her up. Her arms would be strapped down with leather thongs.

The circumstances of such births were the opposite of everything American women had come to expect about having a baby. The doctor, who in the United States would be napping on a parlor sofa while he waited for the woman to finish dilating, was awake and alert to monitor the drug dispensing, while the mother-to-be, who would normally be working herself into a sweat, was floating in oblivion.

After the delivery, Sister Mary Louise Peters, the head nurse, in a white cap and dress, would bathe and clothe the infant and present the child on a pillow to its groggy mother. In one account, recalled in *McClure's Magazine* in 1914, Sister Mary Louise handed a baby to its disbelieving mother and said:

"Here is the handsomest boy in the clinic. Do you know him?"

"I want to see my own child," the woman replied.

"She wants to see her own child," Sister Mary Louise devilishly said to the doctor. "What shall we do about it?"

"Give him to her," he said.

Scopolamine wasn't new. The drug is an alkaloid of belladonna, a poisonous plant that has red, bell-shaped flowers. Ancient Greeks used it to help men forget their "burdensome engagements." But scopolamine was an unstable agent that was difficult to calibrate if not stored or handled properly. The doctors at the University of Freiburg had figured out a way to solve that problem, although they ruled out the use of scopolamine for general surgery because too much of it was needed in conjunction with morphine to totally anesthetize the patient. In lesser doses, however, they found it to be just right for childbirth. Scopolamine made the mother lose her inhibitions, which is a good thing during labor—especially in an era of social and physical corseting. But she also could feel helpless and become highly excited, which is why the doors were padded.

Word of Twilight Sleep spread across the globe. Women from India, Russia, South Africa, and North and South America came to savor the new, oblivious style of childbirth. They couldn't praise it enough. Women in the United States—and about a decade later, their British counterparts—had begun equating the elimination of birth pain with their political liberation and right to vote. American socialites published books and pamphlets about

Twilight Sleep and sponsored lectures, tours, and rallies about the method, including one at Gimbel's department store in New York City in November 1914. There, amid the fancy clothes, Twilight Sleep proponents displayed healthy "Freiburg babies" and said the method should be available beyond the five American hospitals that had just begun offering scopolamine-morphine injections.

"I experienced absolutely no pain," Frances X. Carmody, the first American woman to travel to Freiburg, just four months earlier, said at the store rally. "An hour after my child was born I ate a hearty breakfast. At night I got out of bed, and, following the doctor's advice, put on my slippers, walked to a couch across the room, and lay down. The third day I went for an automobile ride. My baby today is getting on fine. I never experienced any ill effects from the drug the doctor gave me. The 'Twilight Sleep' is wonderful, but if you women want it you will have to fight for it, for the mass of doctors are opposed to it."

Some medical studies had found that Twilight Sleep was not only safe but helpful in deliveries because the drugged women relaxed into their contractions, aiding dilation and making it less likely that the doctor would have to use forceps. (Many believe the same premise holds true today with epidurals.) But American obstetricians were still alarmed. They knew that Twilight Sleep newborns did not always breathe immediately, that some mothers still felt the pain, and that there was great risk of stalled labors and postpartum hemorrhaging. On top of that, they were aware of the seedy underside of Twilight Sleep, the side that the injected women did not remember: the thrashing, the helmets, straightjackets, and wrist cuffs mothers were forced to wear for protection. After the method migrated to the United States, residents of one New York neighborhood near a Twilight Sleep hospital reported hearing "objectionable" noises in the middle of the night. One doctor said his screaming patient could be heard four floors below.

However, Twilight Sleep's most strident supporters complained that American doctors were just being stubborn and sexist and that they wouldn't adopt the method because it was not their idea. So women took matters into their own hands, opening Twilight Sleep facilities in major cities such as New York, Chicago, and Boston. Frances Carmody herself founded one such hospital in Brooklyn. But her devotion to Twilight Sleep literally consumed her life. Tragically, Carmody bled to death after her second Twilight Sleep delivery, in August 1915. Her husband denied that the drugs had anything to do with the hemorrhage, even though excessive bleeding was an established side effect of scopolamine-morphine. Still, one would think her high-profile death—combined with growing animosity toward all things Teutonic on the eve of World War I—would have mitigated the method's popularity.

The opposite happened. Remarkably, Twilight Sleep went mainstream. As more and more women aspired to give birth the way society women had made fashionable—a common pattern throughout history—even skeptical doctors in traditional lying-in hospitals succumbed to consumer demand. And then they took it one step further. In America, doctors, who could now write off their patient's delirious cries, ignore them for hours, and treat them roughly without consequence, made Twilight Sleep practically mandatory. By the early 1930s, hospital delivery procedures were so bound up with inhaled or injected drugs that mothers almost always gave birth while heavily medicated. (This was true of my grandmother's deliveries in the 1940s, and it remained true when my mother gave birth to me in 1969.) In fact, Twilight Sleep stubbornly persisted as standard practice in some American hospitals as late as the 1970s. In the meantime, women who wanted to be conscious during birth had to work hard to find an obstetrician, or a maternity facility, that would allow her to remain awake and alert.

NATURAL CHILDBIRTH

Lenore Pelham Friedrich's journey to have a drug-free birth was extreme, especially for its day. In 1933, this college-educated woman living in New York City had moved to a farm, where she saw many animals give birth peacefully and stoically, something she believed she, too, was capable of. Because her first three children had been born while she was under ether—struggling to regain consciousness was worse than the idea of any pain for her—she was determined to have her next delivery naturally.

"I was going to have it straight," she said, "preferably at home. But this was impossible. The well-trained doctors in the country simply did not deliver babies. [They had more important things to do.] The ones who went about to the farm women seemed to me less competent than what I wanted. In the city. . . it was equally impossible. The obstetrician flatly refused. 'I don't like to see people suffer' was his reason for insisting on anesthesia." And so, on the eve of World War II, Mrs. Friedrich packed her bags and headed to Switzerland, to have a baby overlooking Lago Maggiore, in a hospital where, when she told the doctor she did not want anesthesia, he told her it was never given.

Meanwhile, in England, obstetrician Grantly Dick-Read was writing that delivering a baby should feel like "a normal and natural defecation," and blamed fear and tension for women's suffering during labor. He believed that if he could reduce anxiety through education and support, birth could become a positive, healthy experience.

Dick-Read's ideas were not necessarily new. Throughout the nineteenth century, European and American physicians speculated that civilized people had more complex nervous systems than "savages" and therefore were more susceptible to pain. Doctors during the 1800s had compared lower-class people to animals, which, they said, lacked the sensibility to hurt in labor; only intelligent women bracing for pain actually felt it. But Dick-Read's controversial message was one that women such as Lenore Pelham Friedrich wanted to hear. Throughout the 1940s and '50s, his views gained momentum in the United States and Europe, even inspiring another doctor, Fernand Lamaze of France, to formulate his own method for drug-free births.

Marjorie Karmel, an inquisitive American graduate of Bryn Mawr living in Paris in the mid-1950s with her husband, Alex, was drawn to Lamaze's practice for her first pregnancy, one that would revolutionize childbirth. Her story begins with birth preparation classes taught by Lamaze's assistant, Mme. Cohen, who guided the couple through six ninety-minute training sessions, two weeks apart, in the middle of her own apartment parlor.

Cohen told the Karmels that pain and body functions are controlled by the cerebral cortex, which is why she would be "training muscles, yes, but that will be the smallest part of your work. Most of the time you will be working on your brain, developing its inherent capability to control your body and suppress pain—in a word, conditioning it to enable you to do what you have to do to have a truly painless childbirth. That is why we don't call our system 'natural' childbirth. The final result should be better than nature."

Karmel was told to lie on her back on a table, and alternately raise her legs as high and as slowly as she could and then lower them. She then was instructed to hold her arms at a right angle to her body and swing her legs up to meet them. This, Cohen said, would help with pelvic floor elasticity. Next, Karmel was to tense her left leg and right arm at the same time, while the right leg and left arm were to be totally relaxed.

The next big exercise was in breathing, the most famous of the Lamaze techniques. As instructed, Karmel inhaled slowly through her nose, keeping her lips pursed. She exhaled slowly and silently through her mouth. She practiced doing this in a rhythm of fake contractions coming at a four-minute clip. The exercise made her dizzy and she said as much to her instructor.

"You're not accustomed to so much oxygen," Cohen said. "When you practice you must be sure to rest before you stand up. Otherwise you may find that you feel faint."

At the next class, Karmel learned how to massage just beneath the belly to soothe the tense muscles. That, combined with the breathing, was supposed to help alleviate the pain. "We suspect that much of the pain of labor is caused by the fact that the extraordinary activity of the uterus exhausts the supply of oxygen in the blood," Cohen told the Karmels. "There may be a chemical reaction resulting from this, an accumulation of toxic substances that causes pain and might be responsible for the sort of cramp that many women experience as an unending state of contraction."

That all made sense to Karmel. Except, why did she have to breathe rhythmically?

"The brain can never be aware of all the sensations that are constantly being sent to it," Cohen explained. "Whenever the brain is engaged in an activity, it shuts out many of the sensations that are sent to it." In other words, the laboring woman would be so busy relaxing this, tensing that, and counting her breath, that she'd be too busy to feel the throes.

When it was time for Karmel to deliver her first child, a son, she went to the clinic with her husband—he was allowed to stay for the birth—and labored for hours in a dimly lit room as midwives fed her tea and mashed potatoes. Cohen arrived with Lamaze only near the end of labor, when Karmel was in the most intense and painful stage. Cohen turned on all the lights and sponged cold water on Karmel's face to keep her concentration sharp. She told her to breathe and relax and directed Karmel to give herself a fluttering fingertip massage on her own belly. Then she gave her a glucose shot to boost her strength.

97

"In a few minutes the pain stopped and my control returned," Karmel said. "The contractions regained strength and shape and I was able to stay on top of them. But there was very little time in between, and I was exhausted."

Karmel also took some oxygen from a plastic mask and felt the intensity of the contractions. "It took all my concentration, even with Mme. Cohen directing me, to remain in control."

Suddenly, as she entered the pushing phase, Karmel felt extremely nervous and was momentarily suspended in a state of not knowing what to do. Then she shouted, "*Ça vient!*" (Here it comes!) Staff pulled the pillows out from under her, put her legs in stirrups, and cheered her on to push. "It was an unbelievable sensation, not at all painful but somewhat terrifying," she said later. Her second and third children were born in New York, also without pain medication.

Karmel chronicled her experience in a 1959 best-selling book, *Thank You, Dr. Lamaze,* which legitimized the techniques across the Atlantic and helped change the culture of medicated births through the 1960s and '70s. But by the 1980s, women had begun to realize that not everyone was equally good at mastering the breathing and relaxation techniques. All of that huffing and puffing was making some women dizzy—and they were still feeling pain. And so, as bellbottoms gave way to big hair, natural birth methods gave way to the epidural.

THE MIGHTY EPIDURAL

At Brigham and Women's Hospital, when the anesthesiologist arrives, he tells the pregnant woman to sit sideways on the bed and then bend forward as much as her enormous belly will allow. The woman follows orders and tightens as he swabs cold disinfectant on her bare lower back and then inserts a needle between her vertebrae. "Ouuuuch!" she cries, drawing the word into two syllables that increase in pitch as she buries her head in her husband's chest for support. The anesthesiologist connects a tube that will deliver the numbing agent bupivacaine, via automatic pump through her spine, during labor and delivery. The effect is quick—the sensation of dead weight fills her legs and abdomen. She remains awake but relaxed as the nurse helps her lie down in an adjustable bed at the same facility where, 158 years earlier, Catherine Fisher had become the first patient in any American maternity hospital to receive an anesthetic; she, of course, was unconscious for the birth.

Today the vast majority of American women call for the needle in the back when pain becomes too intense. This method of administering pain relief was pioneered in 1898 by German doctor Karl August Bier, who injected cocaine into his assistant's lower back. To test whether the assistant, Dr. Hildebrandt, was numb, Bier

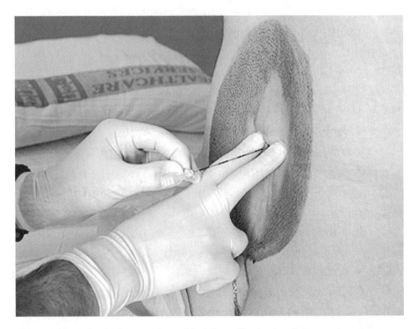

An anesthesiologist inserts the epidural needle during labor. (Photo by Patti Ramos)

pulled on the man's pubic hair, yanked his testicles, hit him in the shins with a hammer, and singed his thighs with a cigar. Hildebrandt felt only vague sensations of being touched. But the next morning, bruised and burned, he awoke with horrible vomiting and headaches, a condition known as the post-spinal headache. The large needle they had used allowed a small amount of spinal fluid to seep out of the dura, a thin membrane that surrounds the spinal cord and brain. When the fluid level drops, the brain can sag, pulling on connective tissue. The result: throbbing head pain.

Even in the 1970s, epidurals were still imperfect. The drug doses were so high that mothers could be numb up to their necks, making it difficult to breathe and causing potentially lethal heart problems. Sometimes the epidural accidentally was injected into a blood vessel, rather than the epidural space, a problem that can cause toxicity. That, too, sometimes led to deadly cardiac arrhythmias.

By the 1980s, half the women giving birth at Brigham and Women's were still not choosing to have an epidural, in part because of the injection's spotty record and in part because natural-birth activists told women that epidurals would lower a baby's IQ, prevent breast-feeding, and inhibit developmental milestones. None of which is true, according to Dr. William Camann, director of obstetric anesthesia at the hospital.

Today, smaller needles mean less chance of a headache, and the smaller dosage of anesthesia numbs the woman only from the waist down. Because every person's epidural tolerance is different, some need a boost of the pain medicine, while others become too numb and need the level reduced. Regardless, the woman remains completely conscious—though often she feels relaxed enough to nap during labor.

God's gift to women? Perhaps. But once again, there are drawbacks. Women hooked up to epidurals are more likely to need artificial stimulation, such as Pitocin, to keep contractions strong. They are also more likely to have their blood pressure drop; develop a fever; and have difficulty passing urine, and so are regularly catheterized. Being unable to feel from the waist down makes pushing difficult, and there is a greater risk of needing forceps or a vacuum to complete the job. Though research has shown that epidurals do not raise the likelihood of a cesarean, there is controversy surrounding the issue. One study has shown that epidurals increase the likelihood of the baby presenting in the posterior position—in other words, not fully rotated. Such a presentation *does* lead to higher cesarean rates.

Nevertheless, epidurals have a virtual lock on hospital pain relief—in the United States, anyway. Somehow, women all over the rest of the globe manage to give birth without them. In Japan, the epidural rate is in the single digits, although that may change: A pregnant Japanese celebrity recently condemned the country's obstetric system and told women they should go to the United States for more powerful drugs. In the UK, women at the peak of a contraction can reach for a mask and inhale nitrous oxide, or laughing gas. They also use TENS, transcutaneous electronic nerve stimulation, in which a handheld device the size of a camera sends buzzing impulses through wires taped to one's back. The impulses, which some women find annoying, are supposed to tell the brain to release natural opiates and endorphins.

In the Netherlands, where home birth is popular, epidurals decidedly are not. "The Dutch really believe birth is not risky; it is a physiological process," says Raymond DeVries, an American professor and author who has studied their approach to birth. Dutch obstetricians don't offer epidurals because such pain relief is not part of the natural process. But there also that might change. "They are considering moving to a more market-driven system," DeVries says of the Dutch government, "so that if a woman asks for an epidural at a clinic, she can get one."

Although studies have shown that women in the last weeks of pregnancy have a greater tolerance for pain, their ability to cope varies widely depending on their cultural attitudes surrounding birth, rather than any innate differences among peoples. In North America and increasingly throughout Europe and Australia, having a baby is viewed as a medical procedure in which many things can go wrong. Pain relief is so socially acceptable that it is virtually expected. Even if a woman is considering forgoing drugs, it's easy for her to be convinced otherwise during labor. When the nurse first pokes her head in the labor room and says, "Do you want your epidural now?" a mother-to-be might think, *I can handle the pain— women have been doing this for hundreds of thousands of years.* An hour later, when her brow is sweaty and she's doubled over with contractions, the nurse comes back. "Do you want your epidural now?" She hates this nurse. She loves this nurse. "Give it to me. Fast," she says, from somewhere deep in her throat. The busy nurse on a twelve-hour shift smiles, calls in the anesthesiologist, and moves on to the next patient. Soon the laboring woman reclines comfortably in bed, talks on the phone, watches a movie, and waits for the baby to come. She is not screaming for the nurse, pacing up and down the hall. She is not cursing, grunting, or moaning. She is quiet. She is a good patient. And she's happy. As is the nurse.

"Why do they push epidurals?" asks Kate Bauer, executive director of the National Association of Childbirth Centers. "It makes the patient easier to manage. At the root of everything, there's money to be made. I'm sure many think they're doing a great service to women by offering the epidural and relieving them of pain, but it also helps them to cut back on the nursing. You've gone from the human touch to this: Give them the epidural and watch the monitor."

Certainly, epidurals have taken the work out of labor—for most involved—and replaced chants, herbs, and breathing techniques with a kit and a power button. But just as Twilight Sleep erased the true experience of childbirth for a generation of women, epidurals may be doing much the same thing. And almost no one is complaining.

5 THE CESAREAN SECTION

FIVE HUNDRED YEARS ago, in a little Swiss town, a woman labored for days, to no avail. The thirteen midwives who had been called in to assist could not help. Her desperate husband, an illiterate pig-gelder, approached the local authorities and asked permission to slice open her abdomen to retrieve the baby. After first saying no, they finally said yes. And so Jacob Nufer went about his dangerous business, delivering a large healthy son. Not only did both patients survive, but the child lived to be seventy-seven and the wife had several more children, including twins, all vaginal births.

Although this story was not recorded until some eighty-two years after it took place, the tale is believed to be the first written record of a mother and child surviving a cesarean. Today, Nufer's dramatic surgical feat has become such a routine operation that nearly one out of every three babies in developed countries arrives by cesarean section. One of the highest C-section rates on earth is in the Brazilian city Rio de Janeiro, where 90 percent of wealthy women would rather pay for the operation than put their vaginas at risk. Cesareans have become so commonplace that we refer to the discreet six-inch scar as a "bikini cut." The pregnant women who schedule surgery even if there's no medical reason for it are "too posh to push."

Before the surgery became routine in the twentieth century, attendants had few other means to extract a stuck fetus. One option was to kill the fetus and remove its body bit by bit through the vagina. If the baby's foot or arm was leading the way down the birth canal, the attendant might dismember the fetus inside the mother and then lay its body parts out on a table to make sure nothing was left behind. The procedure was called an embryotomy.

If the fetus was stuck in the more common head-down position, the attendant could perform a craniotomy, the equally horrible procedure described earlier. A seventh-century text by Paulus Aegineta explains how the mother would be tied to a bed with ropes across her chest, and a woman on each side of her would hold her thighs up and apart. Another helper would separate the outer opening of the vagina, while yet another would manually open the cervix, if necessary, and insert a hook, grabbing on to any part of the baby it could reach. Another hook would grab hold just opposite the first so the baby could be pulled straight out. Old Hindu texts talk about severing the head and pulling it out. If shoulders were stuck, the arms would be cut off. As violent as it sounds, the baby often was already dead before such desperate measures were taken. If left too long in the womb, the decomposing fetus would have lethally poisoned the mother. Some doctors, however, advocated leaving the fetus to die so it could begin disintegrating, thereby making it easier to extract.

Craniotomy was a painful and emotionally agonizing procedure for all involved. American doctor Charles Meigs admitted having to take breaks during a tedious craniotomy that dragged on for hours. In another case history from 1840, the doctor described the craniotomy he performed on a woman with a pelvic brim of only 1.5 inches. He began drilling the fetal skull at midnight and didn't finish removing the body until 2:00 p.m. the next day, when he had to be carried home in a sedan chair. The woman, he said coldly, was "fine."

There was great moral and religious debate about craniotomy. The Catholic Church did not like the procedure because it meant certain death for the fetus, often before it could be baptized. Instead, the Vatican preferred cesareans, even though that often meant the mother would die.

In 1733, doctors had asked theology specialists at the Sorbonne in Paris whether it was religiously acceptable to sacrifice the mother by performing a most likely lethal cesarean if the baby could not be vaginally delivered. The scholars said the conflict of having to choose which one should live—woman or child—favored the baby because it had to be baptized, or else its soul would be stuck in purgatory.

In his 1930 encyclical, Pope Pius XI declared that doctors could not take a baby's life to save the woman's. After the pope's directive, cesarean rates spiked, as indeed did maternal mortality, since the operation was still far from safe.

Not all doctors made the decision based on religion. Practicality was also a factor. If the mother's pelvis was too small, piecemeal extraction might be impossible anyway, in which case, cesarean was the only option. Other doctors favored craniotomy, either because the fetus had stopped moving and was presumed dead, or because they theorized that the unborn had no pain or feeling.

Because neither cesarean nor craniotomy was ideal, doctors were always searching for an alternative. One breakthrough, if it can be called that, came in 1777, when French surgeon Jean René Sigault sawed through the pubic bone of Madame Souchot, a three-foot, eight-inch, rickety thirty-year-old who was about to give birth. None of her four earlier pregnancies had ended with a live baby. Knowing all this, as well as the fact that her pelvis was only 2½ inches wide when measured on the diagonal, Sigault experimented with a procedure he had practiced only on animals and criminals. Shortly after midnight, with no anesthesia and by the light of a candle, Sigault cut through her clitoris, through the labia, and into the urethra. He then inserted his left index finger behind the symphysis—the middle of the pubic bone—and divided the cartilage,

widening her pelvis by about 2½ inches. He ruptured her membranes and delivered a healthy breech baby boy. The mother also
survived, though not without serious complications. She was rendered permanently incontinent and even years later needed help
to walk. Without the support of the bony pelvic girdle, which remained separated, her uterus prolapsed and her vagina became
inverted, hanging outside of her body, between her legs. Women
who'd had this procedure would insert ball-like pessaries, made
of everything from wax to potatoes, to plug their organs inside.

Between 1777 and 1858, there were fifty-six documented
cases of the operation, called a symphyseotomy. A third of the
mothers and more than half of the infants involved died. Although
Sigault had won accolades for that first recorded "successful"
symphyseotomy with Madame Souchot, her suffering made him
feel less sure of the procedure's merits, and he eventually recommended cesareans instead.

Symphyseotomy was never popular in the United States;
about forty were performed at Johns Hopkins before 1915, after
which doctors switched to cesarean sections. However, the pubic
bone cutting endured in Ireland, Africa, and Italy. Symphyseotomy
is still done in poor countries where women don't have access to
a cesarean. In 1991, twenty symphyseotomies were performed in
Nigeria's St. Luke's Hospital.

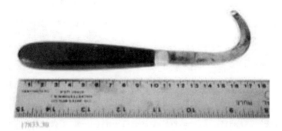

*A knife for cutting through the pubic symphysis, the cartilage that hinges
the two halves of the pelvis together, to widen the birth canal. (Courtesy the
Mütter Museum)*

Aware of the shortcomings of the symphyseotomy, doctors developed another procedure to deliver a stuck fetus: They began to cut the cervix. In 1791, Dr. Thomas Archer of Maryland asked his attending midwife to hold a candle so he could see what he was doing, and without warning either woman, pulled out a common spear-pointed lancet and made three two-inch incisions to widen the neck of the uterus to get the baby out. The patient reportedly recovered several weeks later. For emergencies, cutting the cervix remained an option far longer than the symphyseotomy, continuing well into the twentieth century, especially in forceps deliveries when obstetricians did not wait for full dilation. Cutting the cervix seems crude, but when Dr. Archer resorted to the desperate method, he probably did not know of any cesareans in which the mother survived.

In Europe, the number of cesareans remained low until relatively recently when U.S.-style obstetric practices burst through the dams of midwife-loving countries. Since the early 1990s, England's cesarean rate has doubled to 22 percent, the same as Canada's. In Italy, home of the Roman Catholic Church with its long history of surgically removing an imperiled fetus in order to baptize it, the rate is about 35 percent. Central and South American rates are also running high: 36 percent in Mexico and 40 percent in Chile. Now a record 29 percent of American-born babies arrive by C-section, making the operation more common than the appendectomy or the tonsillectomy.

Although vanity, convenience, and precautions for the fetus are leading more women to avoid the unpredictability of vaginal births, a cesarean can still have deadly consequences, and serious side effects. A baby born by cesarean is at risk of being nicked by the scalpel, and there is an increased likelihood of difficulties with initial breast-feeding attempts; pain, which lingers after the surgery, can suppress milk production. The mother also is more prone to develop postpartum depression, infertility, and placenta abnormalities in future pregnancies, as the placenta can have difficulty implanting around the scar. Three such abnormalities can lead to dangerous and possibly fatal hemorrhaging: Placenta previa, in which the placenta implants over the cervix; placenta acreta, in which it implants through the uterine tissue; and placenta abruption, in which the placenta pulls away from the uterine wall before it should. Obstetricians are observing such cases more and more among Mormon women, a tragic consequence of cesareans in a population that produces many children.

Yet a C-section, when performed under the proper conditions, is remarkably safe—even, occasionally, when performed under less than optimal conditions. In 2002, a forty-year-old Mexican woman went into labor with her ninth child. Labor was not going smoothly, and, having lost one baby in childbirth before, the woman was determined that this one would live. In her remote dirt-floor home, alone, with no electricity or running water, she drank three glasses of liquor. Then, equipped—as the pig-gelder had been—with a kitchen knife as well as experience in slaughtering animals, she gave herself a crude cesarean section, eventually opening her abdomen after three attempts.

She delivered a healthy child, a boy, who breathed right away. Before losing consciousness, she ordered one of her other children to find a local nurse, who arrived to close the incision with an ordinary needle and thread. Only later was the mother taken to the hospital in Oaxaca, eight hours away. The surgery is recorded in medical journals as the first time mother and child survived a self-administered C-section.

It's not surprising that the tales of the sixteenth-century Nufer family and the contemporary Mexican woman seem almost mythical. Cesareans have always been the stuff of myth. Many gods were said to be C-section babies, including Asclepius (god of healing), Dionysus (god of fertility and wine), and the handsome Adonis. Even Buddha was supposedly born through a slit in his mother's side. Many cultures believed babies who survived such a surgical birth held special powers or abilities. Take the Persian tale of Zal's wife, Rudaba, who, when pregnant with an enormous child, was given hyoscyamus, a poisonous herb that can relieve pain and cause unconsciousness. She fell into a death-like sleep, and a Zoroastrian priest cut from her abdomen the Persian Hercules known as Rustam.

Even the naming of the cesarean involves a myth.

There is a common assumption that the cesarean section was named after Julius Caesar who, legend has it, was cut out of his mother's womb. However, that act at that time would have surely killed her. Caesar's mother, we know, survived his birth and died only after he invaded Gaul. Another theory—one that is trickier to follow—is that Numa Pompilius, the second king of Rome, decreed around 700 BC that a fetus had to be surgically

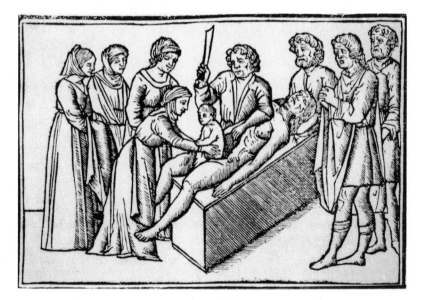

The purported birth of Julius Caesar, as depicted in Suetonius's Lives of the Twelve Caesars, 1506 woodcut. (Courtesy the Wellcome Library)

removed from the womb if its mother was dead or dying. His decree was part of the *Lex Regia*, the royal law, which later became known as the *Lex Caesare*. Also, because the surgery was a "grand" operation, as grand as a caesar, many believe cesareans are therefore named generically after the rulers of Rome. In fact, until the First World War, Germans called the operation a *Kaiserschnitt*, after the ruling kaisers.

Over time, all of these details blurred. Julius became the most famous caesar Rome produced, and the legend of his surgical birth was perpetuated, especially through art. Paintings depicted Caesar being pulled out of a bloodless gaping hole in his mother's abdomen. Early paintings depict women doing the cutting for his birth. Later artwork placed the knife in the hand of a man, reflecting how males were beginning to muscle out women as attendants in the birthing room, especially in complicated cases.

Despite the prevalence of these myths, during the sixteenth and seventeenth centuries, C-sections were rare, performed exclusively when all hope was lost. An Italian Renaissance text instructed surgeons to attempt the operation only on strong, courageous women, and with strong, courageous attendants to hold them down. After careful examination, the surgeon would draw a line about six inches long to mark the incision, then slice vertically through the abdominal rectus muscles (what some now try to tone into a "six-pack") before gingerly cutting into the uterus. The baby and placenta were pulled out; a sponge was used to mop up the mess; and the bleeding was supposed to be stopped with the help of a stew of artemisia, agrimony, betony, mallow, dried roses, flowers of pomegranate, birthwort, sedge, and sweet-smelling bulrushes. The woman then had a linen pessary, soaked in rose oil and egg yolk, inserted in her vagina three times a day in the summer and twice a day in the winter, to absorb draining blood and other fluids. (It's not clear why pessaries were changed more often in the summer.) The surgeons also may have thought the concoction prevented infection, the causes of which were unknown at the time.

Miraculously, several women in the eighteenth century survived the operation. Alice O'Neal was one of them. The thirty-three-year-old farmer's wife from Charlemont, Ireland, already had several children, but had never experienced a labor like the one she endured in 1738: It went on for twelve days, a parade of desperate midwives failing to deliver the child. Finally, they called Mary Donally, a midwife known for extracting dead fetuses, for by this time, they assumed the baby had perished. Although the record doesn't say, Donally may have offered O'Neal a little whiskey before slicing into the woman's abdomen with a razor and then cutting into the uterus, making a six-inch incision on the right side of the navel. She removed the stillborn, placenta, and membranes, and held the wound together with her hands while a neighbor fetched silk thread and a tailor's needle. She then dressed the wound with egg whites. The mother survived, albeit with a ventral hernia—the protrusion of an organ through a part of the abdominal wall which, in her case, had been weakened by the surgery. Less than a month later, she was able to walk a mile.

But the rare woman who made it through the agony and potential shock of the surgery faced other troubles, primary among them infection. In 1785, surgeon John Aitken of Scotland, incorrectly believing that air entering the abdominal cavity caused infection, advised that cesareans be performed with the woman's body submerged in tepid water. Also, until the operation became more standardized in Europe and America in the late 1800s, incisions were imprecise. Most were vertical, some extending as high as the rib cage, causing the intestines to spill out. Some were diagonal. There were surgeons who would make multiple cuts until they got it right. The person performing the operation would yank the baby out as quickly as possible by the foot, believing its head was at risk of being clamped down on by a contracting uterus. Sometimes the placenta was left alone, allowed to pass through the birth canal on its own. Or the placenta might be accidentally cut during the uterine incision, leading to a fatal hemorrhage.

In Paris between 1787 and 1876, no woman is known to have survived a cesarean. In 1793, there was one C-section in England, believed to be that country's first that the mother survived. Jane Foster had once fallen off a loaded cart, and the wooden wheels, transporting heavy freight, had rolled over her pelvis and broken it. Yet the forty-year-old managed to get pregnant and carry the baby to term. After three days of labor, however, the baby had not been born. Her physician refused to perform a cesarean, viewing the operation as so risky as to be immoral. Seeking help, he called Dr. James Barlow, who was shocked to find that the opening of the birth canal was so distorted he couldn't get his fingers through. Meanwhile, the mother had stopped feeling contractions the night before he arrived. She was anxious, her breathing rapid; attendants had bled ten ounces from her, a common practice in those days for a variety of ills.

"Indeed, the idea [of a cesarean] seemed so dreadful that I did not urge it much, especially when I recollected that of nine or ten instances in which that operation had been performed, in this country, not one had furnished a voucher of success," Barlow later wrote. "In this forlorn and dangerous situation [Foster] was left to the care of a midwife and desired to make up her mind as soon as possible concerning the operation. On the morning following I was again sent for and found her lingering in the same position. She consented to the operation without the least hesitation." With a little help, he took her out of bed and placed her on a table; propped her up with pillows; cut a 5.5-inch vertical incision through skin, muscle, and uterus; and delivered a dead baby and placenta. Foster made a full recovery.

America's first known successful cesarean happened a year later, in 1794, in a log cabin near Staunton, Virginia. Mrs. Bennet's pelvis was so small that forceps were useless, and, believing she would die anyway, she asked for a cesarean over a craniotomy. The doctor refused to operate, so her husband, Jesse, performed the surgery. His wife, under the influence of opium, was splayed out on a wooden plank spanning a couple of barrels. With one quick stroke—the story seems to have been embellished over time—the father sliced open the abdomen and uterus, delivering a healthy baby girl and the placenta. Before he closed the wound with linen thread, he said, "This shall be the last one" and took her ovaries out, too. Mrs. Bennet recovered.

TECHNICAL ADVANCES

In 1879, a Ugandan healer washed his hands in banana wine and splashed some on the pregnant belly of a woman, who drank the rest and slid into semi-intoxication. Her throat and thighs were pinned down on an inclined bed. One man kept her belly still,

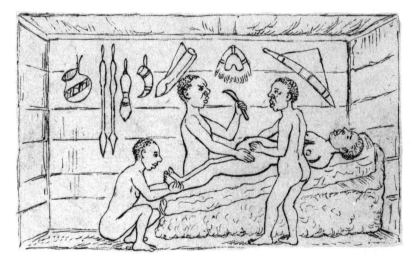

R.W. Felkin, a British traveler to Uganda, sketched the scene of a cesarean. (Courtesy the National Library of Medicine)

while another held her ankles. The healer muttered an incantation and then a shrill cry, and with a knife, he cut through her skin and into the uterus. An assistant used a hot iron to cauterize and minimize bleeding while the healer pulled out the child and the placenta. The assistant struggled to keep the mother's intestines from springing out as the healer massaged the uterus to help it contract. But he did not suture it. And then, instead of using thread or wire, he used iron pins to close the outer abdomen and dressed the area with root paste. Eleven days after the operation, the woman had recovered.

It's a mystery how this woman survived without having her uterus sewn shut. Surgeons had been perplexed for ages over how to close the uterus without causing infection. According to the historical record, in 1769 a French surgeon, Lebas, was the first to stitch the uterus. Although his patient recovered, she suffered from a terrible infection and he was widely criticized. Stitching the uterus led to infection because the thread had to remain inside the woman after the abdomen healed. Some doctors left the suture thread long enough on one end that it would extend outside the abdomen, to be removed later by pulling on it. Others gingerly used one stitch, as if trying not to call attention to the fact that it was there. Yet not to stitch almost always led to a fatal hemorrhage.

In 1876, Professor Eduardo Porro of Italy pioneered a novel way to reduce hemorrhage or infection: He turned cesareans into hysterectomies, believing that if he removed the reproductive organs altogether, less would go wrong. If you think of the uterus as a balloon, the narrowest part, where you blow it up, is the cervix. Instead of trying to piece back together the ripped balloon, Porro merely cut it off at the base, or cervical stump, leaving a smaller wound surface with less bleeding. His first patient for the procedure was Julia Cavallini, a twenty-five-year-old with rickets, in labor for the first time. Her pelvic opening was less than two inches wide. He gave her chloroform and washed his hands in a diluted solution of carbolic acid, and cut her open, removing a healthy baby girl and the placenta. He then cinched the uterus at its base to remove it along with the ovaries and fallopian tubes. He cleaned out her insides with sponges soaked in more carbolic acid and laid some drainage tubes before sewing her up. Cavallini was well in about a month.

Although the church didn't like Porro's approach because it rendered a woman barren, a bishop exonerated him, saying it was acceptable to sacrifice any future children in order to save the existing mother and child. Indeed, the Porro technique dramatically improved the worldwide cesarean survival rate to about 44 percent.

The next advancement came from Germany in 1882, when Max Sanger used silver wire thread to close the uterus. Sanger got the idea to use the silver wire from American doctor J. Marion Sims. Silver is antimicrobial and has been used throughout the ages as a medicinal agent. The Sanger method involved first emptying the bladder, shaving the vulva, and disinfecting the belly and external genitals. He then made a foot-long incision, ruptured the membranes through the birth canal if necessary, and sometimes pulled the uterus out of the body before cutting it open. (Many doctors today pull the uterus out of the abdomen, *after the baby is removed,* to stitch it.) Sanger would remove the child and wait for the placenta to separate from the uterus before pulling that out as well. He then sewed the organ shut with two layers of stitches, followed by suturing the abdomen. Sanger knew how to create a sterile environment and was careful to make sure no fluid from the uterus escaped into the abdominal cavity, even using a waterproof material moistened with carbolic acid around the cervix. His success rate was 80 percent.

Overall, by the late 1800s, the maternal mortality for C-sections was down to 56 percent. Since then, the standardization of sterile procedures, the advent of antibiotics, and the use of lower and smaller uterine incisions have pushed the overall emergency and nonemergency cesarean mortality rate in the United States to .04 percent, compared with .01 percent for vaginal births. As cesareans became less lethal, they also became more common.

SOARING SECTIONS

It's a Friday in 2005, and the anesthesiologists at Brigham and Women's are bracing for a hectic shift of cesareans scheduled every two hours, as well as the usual batch of emergencies that will bump some women into Saturday. By 7:30 a.m., the day shift's first customer, dressed in a hospital gown, waddles into the blindingly lit, chilly operating room. The temperature, set in the low 60s, prevents bacteria growth and keeps the obstetrician from sweating under the blinding lights. The pregnant woman sits on the table, whimpers as an anesthesiologist inserts an epidural needle into her back, and then is helped to lie down. Her arms are splayed and strapped to padded wings. Soon, she is numb from the armpits down. We know this because the anesthesiologist pokes her with a pink plastic cocktail sword from belly button to chest and gets no reaction, even though the patient is wide awake. Meanwhile, a staff nurse is sticking a catheter between the woman's legs, and the obstetrician is using a blue marker to indicate where to cut, along the bikini line, right near the scar from the last cesarean. The mother feels woozy, and the anesthesiologist holds a kidney-shaped bedpan near the patient's mouth in case she vomits, a common reaction to the anesthesia.

The nervous father then enters the room, in full blue hospital scrubs with a cap and mask. He takes a seat on a stool near his wife's head, but it's not easy for his eyes to avoid the mound of flesh at center stage, marked up and smothered in orange antiseptic soap, beneath which their third boy awaits birth. On either side of the operating table, clear plastic saddle bags hang over the edge to catch blood and amniotic fluid. A blue sterile drape effectively separates

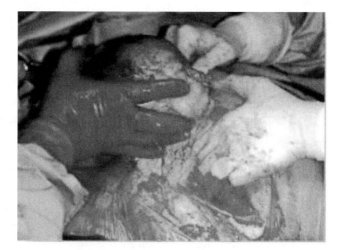

Baby being born by cesarean. (Photo by Patti Ramos)

the woman's face from the rest of her body, and she is connected by tubes of plastic spaghetti to machines that measure her heartbeat and blood pressure and drip fluid into her veins. The woman finally pukes into the pan, and a doctor suctions it up, gives her more oxygen and antinausea medication. Dad coughs nervously, gripping his wife's hand. Mom's eyes are closed tight.

The obstetrician takes a razor—one of about forty stainless-steel instruments lined up on a sterile cart—and carefully begins to navigate scar tissue from the last cesarean. She continues cutting and cauterizing until the uterus is open. Then she thrusts her hands almost elbow deep inside the patient, grabs the baby's head, and begins to tug. The patient's numbed lower body jiggles, jerks, and bounces on the table while the wrestling match with the baby continues. The uterine opening is small by design, so that there is no more bleeding, sewing, and healing than necessary.

At 8:22 a.m., fifteen minutes after the cutting began, the baby emerges. He shrieks and flails as pediatricians carry him to a corner bassinette, wipe him off, and suction amniotic fluid from his lungs. By 8:31, he is wearing a hat, a diaper, and a security ankle bracelet; he's had standard anti-infection drops in his eyes and a shot of vitamin K. He's in Daddy's arms by 8:35, when the surgery team is counting instruments and gauze towels as part of regular safety precautions to make sure nothing is left inside the mother before the uterus is stitched and the abdomen is stapled shut. If all goes as planned, the mother will be home on Monday, nursing the baby and a sore six-inch scar, willing herself not to sneeze or laugh, which just adds to the pain.

In recent decades, as birth rates in developed countries began to drop due to shifting religious beliefs and greater access to contraception, parents decided that they would have just one, two, maybe three children—and they expected each of the progeny to be perfect. Such modern expectations, combined with doctors' fears of malpractice, can lead a woman, if there is any chance of complications, to opt for, or readily agree to, a cesarean. Demographic, medical, and economic changes mean more deliveries are being diagnosed as high risk: Women have been delaying pregnancy until they're older; more of them are undergoing fertility treatments, leading to more complicated multiple births; and medical advances are helping women with chronic conditions, such as diabetes, to carry babies to term.

Women who know in advance that they are having the surgery are probably: carrying twins, past their due date, or have preeclampsia (dangerously high blood pressure, which could lead to convulsions), herpes, diabetes, or a placenta problem. (Before cesareans were a common remedy for placenta previa, the birth attendant might pack the cervix with gauze, seize the foot of the fetus, and pull its buttocks down to cut off placental circulation, hoping the mother did not bleed to death.) And of course, many women schedule a cesarean simply because they had one before and they—or the obstetricians—don't want to risk a VBAC.

Breeches, which constitute about 3 percent of all births, are increasingly born by cesarean. Traditionally, mortality rates for natural deliveries of breech babies had been as high as 10 to 20 percent. Breeches can be tricky to deliver vaginally because the buttocks, knees, or feet are inefficient dilators of the cervix, and labor is often prolonged as a result. Furthermore, women often feel the need to push before the cervix is completely open, which could strangle the fetus. In breech births, the skull is also subject to a more rapid descent than in the births of head-first babies. That could cause brain damage. Although some surveys have found greater incidence of complications with vaginal breech births, a 2005 Norwegian study looked at nearly 400,000 boys, some born breech and the others head first, between 1967 and 1979 and found no difference in intelligence between the two groups as adults.

Although many midwives will deliver breeches, usually trying to turn the fetus first, cesarean deliveries of breeches have become the norm. Between 1970 and 1978 cesarean breech deliveries in the United States jumped from 11.6 percent to 60.1 percent. Today, almost all breeches born in American hospitals are by C-section, in part because the malpractice risk is too great and most obstetricians are no longer proficient in the delicate art of delivering them naturally.

Another, more disturbing condition that could require a cesarean is female genital mutilation. In Somalia, 95 percent of women undergo pharaonic circumcision. In this procedure, the clitoris and labia minora, the two thin folds of skin at the opening of the vagina, are removed, and the labia majora, the outer lips, are sewn closed, leaving an opening so small that a pediatric speculum sometimes has to be used for a gynecological exam. Such mutilation makes vaginal deliveries potentially dangerous, even more so because the average Somali woman gives birth to 7.3 babies. Maternal mortality is 1,100 per 100,000 in that country, making it one of the deadliest places on earth to give birth. Sweden, by contrast, has one of the lowest death rates at 2 per 100,000.

Since the early 1990s, many Somali refugees have been settling in Minnesota, a place vastly different from the home they knew, with very different birthing practices. Somali women, used to large episiotomies to facilitate vaginal birth back home, don't want cesareans. American doctors, of course, dealing with such an unfamiliar condition, would often rather perform a cesarean. At least the doctors in Minnesota would be aware of their patient's circumcision before delivery, allowing for a discussion of the various options. Such planning is a luxury; for despite how common planned cesareans are now in America, the operation regularly is also performed under emergency circumstances.

One of the most common reasons for these unplanned surgeries is "failure to progress," a sort of catchall term that means the baby is not emerging, because it won't fit, it's in a bad position, the contractions aren't powerful enough, labor is taking too long, or the pushing phase is too drawn out, putting the child at risk for a potentially damaging decrease in oxygen intake.

Another typical cause for an unexpected cesarean is because a "nonreassuring" fetal heart rate is detected by the electronic fetal monitor (EFM). These machines, developed from technology that NASA used to monitor astronaut heart rates, were popularized for use in high-risk pregnancies in the late 1960s, replacing the hands-on simple cone-shaped fetal stethoscope. Doctors thought the electronic device's continual monitoring would prevent cerebral palsy and other birth injuries. But in all the years of fetal monitoring there has been no reduction in the incidence of cerebral palsy, which stems from lack of oxygen either at birth or before labor. Many critics, studies, and even obstetricians marvel at the machine's inaccuracy in, on the one hand, detecting trouble; on the other, signaling that the baby is having difficulty when in fact the child is fine. About 15 percent of all laboring women end up with an emergency or "stat" C-section because of the fetal monitor's nonreassuring signals. A 1993 report in the *American Journal of Obstetrics & Gynecology* looked at ten major studies of the monitors and found that a fast or slow fetal heart pattern could not accurately predict how a baby was doing. Konrad Hammacher, a primary inventor of the Hewlett-Packard monitor, a world sales leader with its machines used in forty-five million births within the first twenty-five years, has said doctors shouldn't use an EFM as the focus of care or the basis for a cesarean. However, mothers, and hospitals fearing malpractice litigation, remain lulled by the sense of safety the beeping devices offer. Birth facilities in developing countries are increasingly placing orders for the same reason. It is a standard adage in maternity wards: Doctors get sued for the cesareans they don't perform or don't perform quickly enough. They don't get sued for performing the surgery.

Or so they think.

LONG ARM OF THE LAW

Angela Carder had battled cancer since she was thirteen, losing a leg and half of her pelvis to the disease. Yet she survived, grew up, got married, and got pregnant. Six months into her pregnancy, in 1987, doctors found a large inoperable tumor on her lung. She was hospitalized in the intensive care unit at the George Washington University Medical Center, heavily sedated, her condition deteriorating quickly. Hospital administrators, knowing that the fetus could be technically viable at twenty-six weeks, worried they could be sued for not trying to save the baby. Carder, floating in and out of consciousness, agreed to a cesarean but thirty minutes later changed her mind. Her doctors feared she could die at any time. They talked to their lawyers, who called in Washington-area judge Emmet Sullivan. After hearing three hours of arguments from both sides, Sullivan ordered the hospital to perform the surgery, acknowledging that the baby had about a 50 percent chance of survival, better than if the cesarean was performed at the moment of Carder's death.

"I have an obligation to give that fetus an opportunity to live," said Sullivan, who choked up while stating his decision. "I have ruled."

The baby, Lindsay Marie, died within hours, of "extreme immaturity." Carder, who regained consciousness long enough to know her baby had been taken from her womb and was now dead, wept before she herself stopped living, two days later. They were buried together, the baby swaddled and placed in her mother's arms. The case drew national attention on the contentious issue of court-ordered cesareans. As of 1987, there had been at least twenty-one court orders—nearly 90 percent of applications granted—in eleven American states. The reasons for the court orders ranged from the mother's suspected drug use to her being brain dead or having placenta previa. Eighty-one percent of the women at the center of those court orders were black, Asian, or Hispanic; 44 percent were unmarried; and 24 percent did not speak English as their primary language. All the women were treated in teaching-hospital clinics or were receiving public assistance.

Carder's parents sued the hospital for three million dollars and won an undisclosed monetary settlement in a landmark decision in 1990. The case forced the hospital—with many others following its example—to establish a policy that recognized a pregnant woman's right to control her own medical care.

Lynn Paltrow, the young attorney with the American Civil Liberties Union who argued the case on behalf of Carder's parents, says the number of court-ordered cesareans has been waning since 1990, but similar cases do emerge. Paltrow, now executive director of the New York–based National Advocates for Pregnant Women, believes these cases have more to do with the abortion debate than anything else. "It is about politics and the increasing role of conservative and fundamentalist politicians using technology to promote their ideology," she says.

Still, such court orders are not limited to America.

In 1992, a judge in England allowed doctors at University College Hospital to force a thirty-year-old woman to undergo an emergency cesarean. The woman, identified only as Mrs. S., was a born-again Christian having her third child. She had refused on religious grounds to consent to the operation after being in labor for two days. Doctors thought her condition was serious. She survived the operation, but the baby died.

In 2005, a pregnant woman living in eastern Australia who already had two children by cesarean told her doctor she wanted the third to arrive naturally. The doctor objected, saying it was not safe. And so when the woman failed to show up for her scheduled surgery, the Royal Brisbane and Women's Hospital reported her to child welfare authorities. The hospital said it was only complying with a law requiring medical staff to consider the well-being of the unborn child. The mother, and her case, promptly withdrew from public view.

Yet for every woman having a cesarean because the law or her doctors say she must, there are numbers of others only too happy to schedule one, preferably before her due date.

TOO POSH TO PUSH

Singer Victoria Beckham (a.k.a. Posh Spice) had a cesarean in 1999, another in 2002, and yet another in 2005. Somewhere in between the births of her three sons, the media began to notice a correlation between husband David Beckham's soccer calendar and her due date. Was she actually scheduling the operative deliveries to ensure that he could be there? Or, was Victoria too posh to push? With Madonna, Elizabeth Hurley, Sarah Jessica Parker, and Kate Hudson all having cesareans, the procedure seemed suddenly trendy among the skinny celebrity set.

Elective cesareans have become increasingly popular with wealthy women around the world, from Brazilian beauty queens to Blackberry-toting superwomen who want to schedule delivery for the end of the work week. Some request a cesarean out of fear that, after hours of hard labor, the doctor would call for one anyway. Why not just cut to the chase, so to speak? And then there's always the risk of tearing and incontinence that can result from a difficult vaginal birth. Out of the three million women who have vaginal deliveries in the United States every year, thousands suffer from bladder or anal incontinence, and nearly half of those become sexually dysfunctional. However, cesareans don't necessarily prevent such injuries. The weight of a pregnant uterus can be enough of a stress on the body to cause some of the same damages, which is often temporary.

While the idea of performing cesareans on women even if they don't physically need them seems relatively recent, the practice dates back to the early twentieth century, when well-heeled women cultivated a certain frailty. In 1908, Dr. Franklin Newell of Harvard Medical School believed that moneyed urban women suffered more when having a baby, and he wanted to prevent them from having "nervous breakdowns" by offering the surgery, instead. "It seems to me that this overdevelopment of the nervous organization is responsible for the increased morbidity of pregnancy and labor which is apparent among these women of the overcivilized class," Newell said. "The advocacy of an elective cesarean section for patients who have no pelvic obstruction will undoubtedly come as a shock to many members of the profession."

Newell's idea was especially radical given that C-sections weren't yet totally safe. But the premise of his argument lingers in obstetric units today, where doctors are only half joking when they say that if a woman goes into labor on a Friday (indicating a workaholic control freak), drives a new Volvo (a wealthy intellectual), and has a written birth plan (preconceived notions of how birth should go), she'll end up with an unplanned cesarean, having failed to expel the child on her own. The point here is that there is powerful anecdotal information that says education or level of sophistication seems to lead to higher cesarean rates for such women. Some believe that women who are used to being in charge of every aspect of their lives just can't give in to the natural process that is birth and unconsciously fight it until labor stalls or the pushing phase goes on way too long.

Of course, whether a woman should be able to ask for a cesarean even if there is no medical need for one is the subject of ongoing debate. Plenty of doctors and birth activists believe cesareans should be reserved exclusively for medical necessity. But a 1997 poll published in a European journal found that 33 percent of obstetricians surveyed would choose a cesarean for themselves or their partner, even if it was an uncomplicated pregnancy.

Even more surprising, attempts to limit cesareans in recent years have triggered a backlash from self-described feminists, who just thirty years ago were on the other side of the debate. An article in the *New England Journal of Medicine* in 1999 argued that setting an overall target rate for cesareans would give women less of a say in their own care. And in 1998, a woman wrote in the *British Medical Journal* that pregnant women should have the right to choose how they want to give birth and that limiting that decision proved that "medical and social prejudices against women sidestepping their Biblical sentence to painful childbirth are still with us."

That's certainly not the case in Brazil, where the vast majority of upper-class women demand the surgery and pay for it themselves. In South Korea, where the cesarean rate is 43 percent, women prefer the operation—which they must pay for out of pocket—over vaginal birth because they want to preserve their narrow hips, believe sex will be better, and their baby's intelligence won't be impaired. The more superstitious among them see a numerologist to determine the best day to give birth and then schedule a C-section accordingly. Some critics contend that hospitals, by exploiting women's hopes and fears, are getting rich off the operations, which cost three times more than a vaginal delivery. In Tehran, women delivering in hospitals with male doctors almost always end up with cesareans, due to religiously imposed modesty that prevents women from exposing their genitalia. As for the doctors, cesareans make their hours more predictable.

Should we be outraged? Nancy Wainer says yes.

Wainer, who went from being an average mom to an anti-cesarean activist to a home-birth midwife, wears a fetus-shaped medallion around her neck, teaches childbirth classes in her basement, and announces, on a placard in her front yard, the name and weight of a baby whose birth she recently attended. The first piece of furniture you see when entering her house in suburban Boston is a shellacked wooden birthing stool.

"When they cut me open for my cesarean, I think a tiger jumped in," says Wainer. "I was not like this. It really woke me up."

Wainer was a speech therapist by training who was married to a dentist when, in 1972, she had an unexpected and traumatic cesarean for the birth of her first child. She felt a loss of control, she felt alone—no husband allowed by her side during the surgery—and she was in pain. She also hated the scar and felt she had missed out on the primal female experience of a vaginal birth.

Soon after the cesarean, she and other women who also had had unwanted C-sections began to meet in each other's living rooms. Together they founded a national grassroots cesarean prevention group known as C/SEC, Inc., Cesareans/Support, Education and Concern, a group that later became ICAN, Inc., the International Cesarean Awareness Network. She met with hospital obstetrical staff, imploring them to let mothers keep their babies immediately after the birth and to allow fathers to be present for the operation. (That is also standard practice now unless the woman is under general anesthesia. Most women have epidurals for a cesarean and remain conscious throughout the surgery. General anesthesia is used if the epidural can't be inserted; that can happen if the woman is in so much pain she cannot sit still or if she has a back problem such as scoliosis. Doctors do not allow fathers or other support people to be in the operating room in cases of general anesthesia because when the woman is unconscious, supporting her, they say, is a moot point.)

Although a trickle of hospitals began allowing fathers to view conscious cesareans as early as 1974, an American doctor told the *New York Times* in 1977 why some facilities still resisted the idea. "Having a father in the operating room," he said, "is like having your mother-in-law in the kitchen." Slowly, that attitude changed. By 1978, more hospitals were allowing men in, but usually only if they had been prepped in advance with a cesarean birth class that included slides and words of caution about everything from the unusual noises of the suction machine to how the wound would be closed.

It did not take long, however, for Wainer to realize that making cesareans "more human" was a misguided mission, especially when she believed that as many as 90 percent were unnecessary. "Nobody was focusing on having a normal delivery in the first place," she says of doctors.

Today, most of the pregnant women who seek out Wainer's midwifery services believe they have already had unnecessary cesareans. And they don't want another one. They've come from as far away as Nepal and California in search of this petite woman, hoping for a VBAC, the term Wainer coined when she was writing her 1983 book *Silent Knife: Cesarean Prevention and Vaginal Birth after Cesarean.*

Until the 1990s, once a woman had a cesarean, the chance was very good she'd have to have another, mostly because of a few famous words—"Once a cesarean, always a cesarean"—that Dr. Edwin B. Cragin, professor of obstetrics and gynecology at Columbia University, uttered during a 1916 presentation to the New York Medical Society. At the time, the American C-section rate was less than 1 percent, and the surgery was performed almost exclusively for a contracted pelvis, a condition that wouldn't change from pregnancy to pregnancy. So if the woman got pregnant again, she'd need another section. End of story. As well, into the 1970s, surgeons cut the uterus vertically, a procedure known as the classical incision, which produced a fragile scar that could tear apart during the next birth. So they relied on Cragin's slogan to explain the reason for the repeat surgery.

However, today the cuts are almost always made in the shape of a faint smile along the bikini line, producing a much sturdier scar. Scottsman James Martin Munro Kerr introduced these lower horizontal cuts in the early 1920s, not because the scars were less noticeable—which of course they are—but because they were more medically sound. Dragging the scalpel horizontally just above the pubic bone was easier for the surgeon. He could slice through a much thinner part of the uterus compared with the fibrous upper portion that did much of the work in contractions. The lower incision, Kerr knew, was also easier on the mother. Healing took less time, there was less blood loss, and there was less recovery pain. The scar was also less likely to rupture in a future pregnancy, making it possible for a woman to labor and have a vaginal birth the next time.

Regardless, the lower incisions took decades to popularize, and Cragin's words still haunted maternity wards as cesarean rates steadily climbed. In 1988, the American College of Obstetricians and Gynecologists (ACOG), under pressure from agitated, liberated women like Wainer, issued a landmark opinion supporting vaginal births after cesareans. The decision led to more VBACs and a brief leveling in cesarean rates.

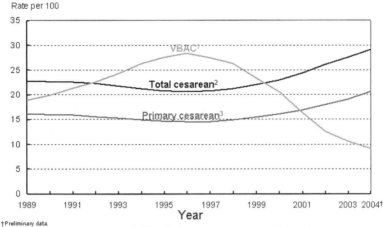

Total and primary cesarean rates and rate of vaginal birth after previous cesarean (VBAC) in the United States, 1989–2004. (Courtesy the National Center for Health Statistics)

But then, in 2002, ACOG reported a new study that showed uterine ruptures in VBACs happened to about 5 in 1,000 women with spontaneous labors and to 24 in 1,000 women whose labors were induced, a fractionally higher rupture rate than previously thought. Within a year, American VBAC rates plunged. More than three hundred American hospitals, worn out by the time and expense of providing necessary backup emergency staff for VBACs, now outright refuse to allow a woman to try a vaginal delivery after a cesarean. In 2004, even American birth centers stopped allowing women to attempt VBACs in their otherwise supportive facilities. The whole situation makes Wainer very angry.

Why, I asked Wainer, do some women who end up with a cesarean get so upset? Why is it difficult to reconcile having a healthy baby with a surgical delivery? Wainer, sitting cross-legged on a wicker chair in her home office, took a sip of her black tea and unfolded her legs. "What if a man can get an erection but can't ejaculate?" she shouted, emphasizing the idea by slapping her hand on her navy blue pants. "He wants the whole experience!"

It was not surprising to see Wainer nearly jump out of her chair in response to the question. Out of all the methods of delivery, cesareans have always been the most emotionally charged. At first, this was because they determined life or death for mother and child. Later, it was because the mother, unconscious and alone, felt robbed of that warm and dreamy moment—the instant her baby is born—partner by her side. Yet today, knowing they can be awake, and flanked by family, if desired, more women are demanding the surgery. More doctors also are insisting on it, leaving those who never wanted the operation, and who never thought they needed it, feeling as stunned as Jacob Nufer's wife must have felt when a knife was plunged into her belly.

6 THE DAWN OF DOCTORS

When forceps became available in seventeenth-century Europe, only members of the all-male barber-surgeon trade could legally use the tools to perform *chirurgery,* as it was called. Having men witness, let alone facilitate, birth after millennia of midwife exclusivity bordered on the scandalous, even if the mother's life was in peril. At first, no one was even sure what to call these men: androboethogynists? Male midwives? Mid-men? Man-midwives? A famous English midwife, angry about the seemingly dangerous and immoral male intrusion into her profession, suggested calling the men "pudendists" after the area of the body in which they were most interested. The French, and later the English, used *accoucheur,* a derivation of the verb "to give birth," a title linguistically problematic because men don't give birth, women do. (*Accoucheur* had come into vogue after Louis XIV chose a man over a female midwife to deliver his mistresses.) Yet it was an English doctor, in 1828, who suggested "obstetrician," the Latin root of which means "to stand before" or, as with the word *obs*truction, "in the way." And in the beginning, that was about all men knew how to do: position themselves at the foot of the bed to catch, snip, or pull.

Barber-surgeons, or man-midwives, were the professional ancestors of obstetricians. Obstetrics, a surgical specialty, is distinctly different from midwifery, which does not legally allow its practitioners to perform cesareans, wield forceps, or apply vacuum extractors. It's easy to see how, from the very beginning of this divergence, midwifery and obstetrics split along gender and philosophical lines.

These early doctors also were different because they were book-trained; they did not have the hands-on practice midwives had. Occasionally, these men might watch a prostitute or destitute woman give birth—no respectable woman would expose herself to a man that way—but such opportunities were rare. Even by 1912, men who graduated from the prestigious Johns Hopkins Medical School in Baltimore likely would have seen only one live birth.

Furthermore, what men taught each other was very different from what midwives passed between generations. One of the earliest midwifery classes men could attend was at the Hotel Dieu in Paris. It was in that hospital that Ambroise Paré (1510–1590), surgeon to the king of France and father of modern surgery, taught his groundbreaking delivery techniques—for better or worse. He reintroduced the ancient art of podalic version, which involves manipulating the fetus in order to pull it out feet first. The maneuver, often used when the shoulder presented first, makes extraction easier because the attendant can grasp the baby's legs. And he revived the inaccurate theory, introduced by Hippocrates, that a woman's pelvis commonly separates (unaided) during birth. But Paré's greatest legacy was having women deliver lying down in bed—a position that made his work easier—rather than on a birth stool, which made the woman's work easier.

In order to attend women while preserving their modesty and preventing embarrassment for all sides, Paré would cover the woman completely with cloth so that he could not see her genitals. Barber-surgeons in England practiced in a similar way, with some eighteenth-century physicians tying a cloth around their own necks like an oversized bib, draping the fabric over their hands and lower bodies, which separated their heads and eyes from their actions. Other barber-surgeons would leave the woman fully dressed, lying on her side and facing away. There would be no eye contact. This side position, more comfortable for women, was used until the early twentieth century, when doctors began preferring their patients, who were often drugged, to be flat on their backs.

Gregoire, an obstetrics teacher in Paris in the century after Paré, taught his students using a basket-weave mannequin that featured a real pelvis taken from a skeleton. The mannequin was wrapped in nude-colored silk, and Gregoire used dead fetuses to show the various presentations and machinations of birth. He also taught his students to use forceps "at random, and [to] pull with great force."

One of Gregoire's students was William Smellie, born in Scotland in 1697. Smellie began his career as a country doctor, getting calls from midwives when a labor was going badly. Once on the scene, he would try to manually rotate the child to allow it to drop into the birth canal, perform a craniotomy, or use a noose to hook the child's head and pull it down if the mother was too exhausted to push. He also bought a pair of French forceps "but found them so long, and so ill-contrived, that they by no means answered the purpose for which they were intended." Smellie eventually moved to London, where he hung a paper lantern outside his house that read "Midwifery taught for five shillings."

He modeled his courses after Gregoire's with one great exception: He brought his male students to the deliveries of poor pregnant women whose desperation to have help trumped any modesty about exposing themselves to a man. (The students had to pay extra to witness these births.) England's earliest hospitals did not accept maternity cases; these women were not sick, after all. And hospitals that specialized in maternity care, British Lying-In, Queen Charlotte's, Royal Maternity, and Middlesex, did not open until later, between 1747 and 1757. As a result, there were plenty of charity cases for these men to watch. Some observers must have been no more than voyeurs. At the end of the War of the Austrian Succession in 1748, a large number of army and navy men began to attend Smellie's lectures. At one delivery, twenty-eight men showed up to watch a birth in a woman's home, causing a near riot in the neighborhood, which rattled Smellie so much that he hurried the case along and broke the child's thigh.

Even those Smellie lessons that involved practice on a "mock mother"—real bones mounted with artificial ligaments and muscles and stuffed with "an agreeable soft substance"—were controversial because his teaching was focused on how to use instruments rather than allowing nature to take its course. He designed a set of wooden forceps that were short and straight, better, most of all, because they didn't clank and scare his patients. He also invented a pair of steel forceps wrapped in strips of leather, again, more for the reason that they didn't make noise than for the purpose of providing better traction. Smellie was secretive about using forceps—even with the woman he was attending—because if something went wrong, the mother might blame the tools, and then the men would have no advantage over midwives. "As women are commonly frightened at the very name of an instrument," Smellie wrote, "it is advisable to conceal them as much as possible, until the character of the operator is fully established."

Smellie, who also operated blindly, told his students to wear a dress to deliveries. There are a couple of ways to interpret that directive. He either wanted his disciples to appear as women, preserving the patient's modesty by tricking her into thinking she was being attended by a midwife; or the dress was just some loose-fitting uniform under which the man could hide his instruments. Dressing as a woman may seem ridiculous, but some barber-surgeons even snuck into birthing rooms, evading the mother altogether so as not to alarm her. In 1658, for example, when a midwife called a barber-surgeon because she was worried that the "birth would come by ye buttocks," the man crawled in and out of the chamber "and it was not perceived by ye lady."

In addition to advocating for dresses, Smellie instructed his students to keep quiet about any birth accident or bad outcome, such as a ruptured uterus, because the competition between the men and midwives was intensifying, and he didn't want such tragedies associated with male attendants. He practiced what he preached. At one birth, as he was fumbling around under the sheets without any direct sight of the woman's vagina or the baby, he accidentally cut the umbilical cord on the wrong side of the ligature, leading to a bloody gush before he could tie it again. The other

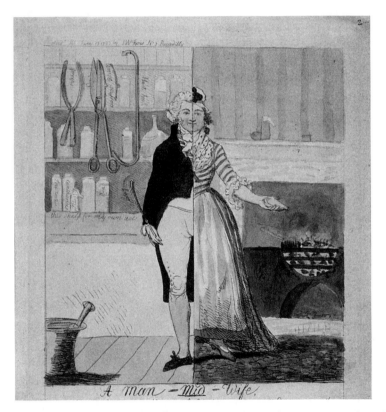

This cartoon engraving by Samuel William Fores, London, 1793, is a literal and figurative depiction of man-midwives, some of whom wore dresses to deliveries. (Courtesy of the Wellcome Library)

midwives in attendance might have been outraged, but the tricky Smellie solemnly announced that it was his way of preventing convulsions in babies.

As Smellie's classes gained in popularity, teaching at least nine hundred men, he became the country's most famous man-midwife. Midwives, who felt threatened by his squad of pupils, ranted about him, as did physicians, who did not see why men would want to associate themselves with such a lowly profession as midwifery.

"I have been told of no less than Eight Women who have died within these few Months under the hands of a Wooden [forceps] Operator," Dr. William Douglas, a main critic, wrote in a 1748 public pamphlet addressed to Smellie. If they had "been of any distinction, you would scarcely have gone on so far."

Douglas had company in his condemnation of Smellie and his minions. In 1760, the respected London midwife Elizabeth Nihell—a rare woman trained at the Hotel Dieu—published an artfully written critique:

> Instead of a child you make use of little stuffed Babies, which have rather amused than instructed your Pupils. This was a wooden statue, representing a woman with child, whose belly was of leather in which a bladder, full, perhaps, of small beer, represented the uterus. This bladder was stopped with a cork, to which was fastened a string of packthread, to tap it occasionally and demonstrate in a palpable manner the flowing of the red-coloured waters. In short, in the middle of the bladder was a wax doll, to which were given various positions. By this admirably ingenious piece of machinery were formed and started up an innumerable and formidable swarm of men-midwives, spread over the town and country.

She went on to complain that men-midwives were nothing more than "broken barbers, tailors or even pork butchers" who "watch the distresses of poor pregnant women, even in private lodgings, where, under a notion of learning the business, they make these poor wretches, hired for their purpose, undergo the most inhuman vexation."

Smellie largely ignored his critics. He died in 1769, but his legacy is profound. He designed a curve in forceps blades to better fit the birth canal, and one of his students, fellow Scotsman William Hunter, established London's first medical school. Hunter advanced the knowledge of how the uterus changes during pregnancy and was Queen Charlotte's physician in the late eighteenth century. Despite Hunter's training, a midwife attended the queen's first birth, while he advised blindly from an adjacent room. It is possible that Hunter helped deliver some of Queen Charlotte's fourteen other children, but having a man attend an upper-class woman in birth was still rare.

One of William Hunter's disciples was William Shippen Jr., who established America's first systemic lectures on midwifery, in Philadelphia in 1765. In these classes, which ultimately banned women, Shippen talked about anatomy, fetal circulation, nutrition, and the use of instruments. He practiced on mannequins and poor patients before wealthy women began to call on him and his colleagues for emergencies. Such women were especially relieved if the man who walked through their door was married.

Because both sexes felt uncomfortable interacting during birth, the mainstream transition from midwife to male attendant was slow. Although the French, in 1801, had refined the ancient speculum so that it offered a full view of the vagina, Americans felt so uneasy with the instrument that the American Medical Association in 1851 recommended against its use, saying it was embarrassing for women and could ruin a doctor's reputation. William Potts

Dewees, who lectured on obstetrics at the University of Pennsylvania in the first half of the nineteenth century, was likewise horrified at the thought of seeing a woman's genitals and taught his students how to perform internal exams without looking. Teaching men how to work in the dark was not just a phenomenon at the University of Pennsylvania. So, too, at Harvard, where Walter Channing, in the 1800s, used a female pelvis and the head of a rag doll to explain fetal positions and how to use forceps. Graduates marched out of the classroom, equipped only with diplomas and the "steel hands" of forceps, into birth rooms where often they would witness the event live for the first time. Worse, they frequently felt compelled to put their tools to work. Channing said a doctor, when called to a delivery, "must do something. He cannot remain a spectator merely, where there are many witnesses, and where interest in what is going on is too deep to allow of his inaction. Let him be collected and calm, and he will probably do little he will afterwards look upon with regret."

Despite the inexperience of male attendants, more and more women began calling for them, though also keeping their God-sibs with them for the birth. This was an era, often testy, when some women clung to the old-fashioned comfort of other females but also were beginning to believe they should have the "more educated" physician there, just in case. Doctors generally didn't like having all these women watching them work and questioning practices.

"The officiousness of nurses and friends very often thwarts the best directed measure of the physician, by an overwhelming desire to make the patient 'comfortable' . . . all this should be strictly forbidden," one doctor wrote in the mid-nineteenth century. "Conversation should be prohibited. Nothing is more common than for the patient's friends to object to [bloodletting], urging as a reason, that 'she has lost blood enough.' Of this they are in no respect suitable judges."

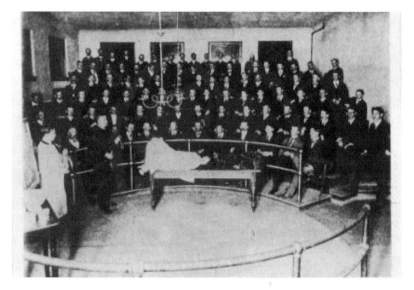

An all-male obstetrics class looking at a female dummy at the Chattanooga Medical College in 1904.

Because obstetric classes in Europe and America had remained all-male for so long, their students learned questionable practices through teachings that were often blatantly sexist. Charles Delucena Meigs (the same doctor who had argued against pain relief in labor) taught the men in his gynecology classes at Philadelphia's Jefferson Medical College that a woman "has a head almost too small for intellect and just big enough for love." When Meigs died in 1869, he was hailed as the dean of American "midwifery." (The term *obstetrics* was not yet used; the field was not a recognized medical specialty in the United States until the early twentieth century.)

Obstetrics remained a male bastion throughout the twentieth century. In 1900, only 6 percent of U.S. doctors were women. Because their numbers were so small, those early female physicians worked hard to portray themselves as more understanding and compassionate, and therefore better than the men. Dr. Mary Dixon-Jones of New York recalled the case of a difficult birth in 1894 during which men urged for a craniotomy but she held out for a live birth. "I spoke up as a woman," she said. "The child must not be destroyed. All the long eight years this woman has had no baby; this will be her comfort, her happiness; it may be her last; we must save it." The mother and child were saved.

Although in recent years the gender balance has finally shifted, the formative years of obstetrics in the U.S. were overwhelmingly dominated by men, beginning with one of the field's best-known physicians, J. Marion Sims.

J. MARION SIMS

In the early 1800s, Sims, an Alabama doctor, was called to a nearby plantation to help Anarcha, a seventeen-year-old slave pregnant with her first child. She had been in labor for seventy-two hours, and there was no end in sight. A doctor overseeing the birth asked Sims to intervene. Sims, fumbling with a pair of forceps with which he had little experience, delivered the child; it was most likely stillborn, the record doesn't say. Five days later Anarcha developed fecal and urinary incontinence, a common result of a protracted labor during which the baby's head presses on the soft tissues of the birth canal, cutting off circulation. The tissue becomes gangrenous and sloughs away until waste leaks uncontrollably through the hole, known as a fistula.

Anarcha's master eventually sent her back to Sims; he had delivered her child, maybe he could heal her, too. Slave women, whose ability to breed made them valuable to plantation owners, were more prone to developing fistulas because their poor diets and a genetic predisposition for lactose intolerance often led to rickets.

Anarcha's was the first fistula Sims had ever seen. But it would not be the last. Incontinence was not just difficult for the slave

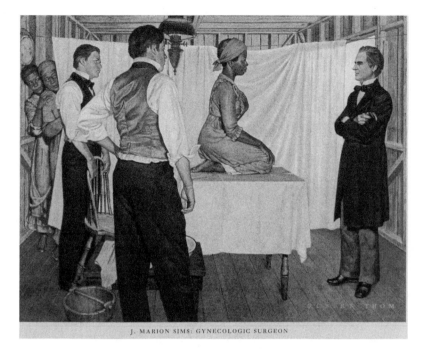

J. MARION SIMS: GYNECOLOGIC SURGEON

In the 1800s, J. Marion Sims, with curved speculum in hand, stands before Anarcha and two physicians. Slaves Betsey and Lucy peered from behind the curtain. Illustration by Robert Thom, from The History of Medicine in Pictures, *1961. (Courtesy Pfizer Inc.)*

women; it repulsed their owners. Two more incontinent slaves, Betsey and Lucy, were sent to Sims to have their fistulas repaired. Sims initially had nothing more than a shoe horn or pewter spoon with which to examine them. He later invented a curved speculum that helped him see the damaged tissue and devised a way to close the fistula without causing infection. He asked a jeweler to make some silver wire to stitch the hole, believing correctly that the metal's antimicrobial properties would help the wound heal.

Sims practiced his grueling technique on slave women for years. Although he claimed the surgery was not painful enough to "justify the trouble and risk" of anesthesia, it is likely that he addicted them to opium. In 1853, Sims set up shop in Manhattan, where upper-class matrons (who would have had access to anesthesia) were so elated that he could cure their embarrassing troubles, they raised money so he could establish the Woman's Hospital of New York City. They also erected a larger-than-life statue of him in Central Park at 103rd Street and Fifth Avenue, where he has been standing on a pedestal, his gaze fixed on the sidewalk, since the 1890s.

Sims's fistula repair—and the slaves' endurance—formed the basis for gynecology as we know it and eradicated the problem in developed countries. However, as many as two million women around the world, most of them in sub-Saharan Africa, still suffer from the birth injury today. We have the knowledge—thanks to the doctor and the slaves—to cure fistulas, but not always the resources.

JOSEPH B. DELEE

Joseph B. DeLee's Chicago-area patients, on the other hand, would have been more likely to suffer injuries from obstetrical swiftness than prolonged labors. DeLee's diary entry from March 11, 1915, sums up his approach: "Delivered boy—forceps—episiotomy (new method worked well)." That method was his "prophylactic forceps operation," an ultimately widely accepted practice in which he used a scalpel to widen the vaginal opening and removed the baby with forceps, regardless of whether or not the child needed assistance emerging.

The episiotomy was an old invention, popularized by Dublin man-midwife Fielding Ould around 1742, to make the exit larger. American doctors became interested in the incision after it was used in the 1870s at the Woman's Hospital in Philadelphia. DeLee picked up on the practice and argued that episiotomies prevented perineal tears that could lead to incontinence and sagging of pelvic floor muscles.

He combined the cutting with forceps use to rescue babies from what he believed was a terrible pounding through the birth canal. He claimed that as many as 5 percent of babies died from head trauma during birth and many others suffered brain damage that, in addition to cerebral palsy, could lead to criminal behavior. At least, such was the thinking at the time. In fact, the clumsy use of forceps was likely the cause for most birth traumas. But DeLee boasted that his procedures—episiotomy and forceps extraction—not only saved the baby from potential trauma, but also left the mother "better than new" after he sewed her up.

None of the more than eight thousand babies DeLee delivered were pushed out by their mothers if he could help it. He would use a modified version of Twilight Sleep during the first stage of labor, and then, as soon as the woman was fully dilated, he would give her an episiotomy and retrieve the child with forceps, sometimes even before the fetus began making its way down the birth canal. In order to do his work, DeLee devised a special bed with stirrups so the woman delivered flat on her back with her feet up.

He argued that birth should be viewed as a disease, one that could be very harmful if not treated and managed by a specially trained doctor. He lectured and wrote articles calling for the abolition of midwives and believed obstetricians were the only ones capable of delivering babies. "The fundamental reason why obstetrics is on such a low plane in the opinion of the profession . . . is just because pregnancy and labor are considered normal, and therefore anybody, a medical student, a midwife, or even a neighbor, knows enough to take care of such a function," he wrote in 1923, by which time he had already amassed a personal fortune and was called the "greatest" American obstetrician of the time. "Once we can convince the profession and the laity that labor has a pathologic dignity, we will be able to draw to this specialty the best minds in the profession."

DeLee's techniques, published in well-read textbooks, were still standard practice in most American hospitals well after his death in 1942. It wasn't until 1983 that the first major study of episiotomies was published. The findings were ominous: Incisions can make the area between the vagina and the anus even more likely to tear as the head emerges; cutting actually weakens the perineum, sometimes causing it to sag. American episiotomy rates, which hovered around 90 percent in the 1970s, had dropped to 39 percent by 1997 and 20 percent by 2000.

GRANTLY DICK-READ

At the height of DeLee's reign, Grantly Dick-Read believed that childbirth did not need nearly as much outside interference. Dick-Read, a young obstetric trainee in the early 1900s and the future founder of the natural-birth movement, was sent out to help a poor woman in labor. When he arrived at her one-room flat in a rough London neighborhood, rain was splashing through a broken window, the space was lit by a candle stuck in a beer bottle, and the woman lay on a decrepit bed, covered with an old black shirt. There was no soap. No towels. Just a jug of water and a basin brought by a kindly neighbor.

Dick-Read, who arrived via bicycle in the middle of the night, was immediately struck by how peaceful the squalid room was. There was no shrieking, no cursing, just a baby emerging, the sight of which propelled him to do what doctors did then. He reached for the chloroform and attempted to cover the woman's face with a mask. She gently refused it. Stunned, he did not force the issue. Later, just as the light of dawn was breaking and he was preparing to leave, he asked her why she did not want the pain relief. She looked around the tiny room and said, "It didn't hurt. It wasn't meant to, was it, doctor?"

The words shocked him. As a child growing up in the English countryside, Dick-Read had always been enchanted by nature and by how animals lived and birthed without complaint. He had always wondered why humans viewed their own birthings as frightening and dangerous. Later, as an army doctor during World War I, he saw both a Belgian woman and a Greek woman "drop a quick one" in the field with little effort and a great deal of joy, seemingly oblivious to the war around them.

Dick-Read eventually theorized that if women were terrified of childbirth, the fight-or-flight reflex would shut down those organs —including the uterus—that are nonessential to fighting or fleeing. With reduced blood flow, the uterus would cramp and cause pain. Because he had also learned yoga-like relaxation techniques during the war from a member of the Indian Cavalry Division, he believed that if women could just "let go," they would experience no pain, have more effective contractions, and therefore have a shorter labor. Likewise, if women were taught what to expect and were supported throughout labor by caring people, there would be no pain.

After the war, working as a junior obstetrician at London Hospital, he began documenting his ideas. Hesitantly, he presented a completed manuscript to the hospital's senior doctors. "Look here old chap," one of them responded. "The truth is we think you really ought to learn something about obstetrics before you start writing on the subject."

Dick-Read later recounted how he had laughed cheerfully to hide his disappointment and promptly put away the paper. Not long after the humiliating incident, he quit the hospital for private practice in the country, where he often found himself at the bedside of laboring women, an audience more receptive to his teachings about relaxation and natural birth.

Although Dick-Read considered using hypnotism and occasionally offered his patients chloroform, his reputation was built on encouraging women to deliver alertly, so as to facilitate what he called "motherlove," or bonding. He also showed women their babies immediately, rather than first cleaning up the newborn and dressing it, as was custom at the time. He believed breast-feeding was essential and encouraged keeping mothers and babies together around the clock. He also thought that if a husband could offer love and support during the birth, then he should be present. Though if he felt the man's own anxiety might worsen the mother's, Dick-Read would not allow him to stay.

As he became increasingly outspoken about his beliefs, Dick-Read angered many who found his natural birth method to be incomprehensible and unscientific. Some doctors asked for scientific proof that his theories were accurate, but Dick-Read had only his personal experiences to offer.

In 1933 he sent his manuscript, *Natural Childbirth*, to a British publisher, Heinemann Medical Books, which agreed to print the work if Dick-Read agreed to pay for it. Which he did. The book, aimed at obstetricians, was the predecessor to his controversial 1942 classic *Childbirth without Fear*, which received overwhelmingly positive reviews, was translated into ten languages, and eventually became a best seller.

"The author maintains that much can be done by ridding women of these fears and his case is stated convincingly," beamed a review in the British medical journal *Lancet*. "One of the most interesting suggestions made is that post-partum hemorrhage is never seen if the mother hears the baby's cry and he suggests that some mechanism exists whereby contractions of the uterus are induced when the mother realizes that the delivery is accomplished." Indeed, more modern science has proven that a baby's cry triggers the rush of oxytocin, a hormone that contracts the uterus and prevents excessive bleeding.

Surprisingly, *Childbirth without Fear* was dedicated to Joseph B. DeLee. Although DeLee delivered his patients in the most unnatural ways, he and Dick-Read did share the view that fear complicated childbirth. Furthermore, Dick-Read was savvy enough to understand that in order to expand his influence and export his ideas to the United States, he needed a prominent doctor, such as DeLee, to legitimize them.

Childbirth without Fear became wildly popular, even in America, where natural births were still practically unheard of. The Maternity Center Association in New York invited Dick-Read to the city to address twenty-five hundred people, including the country's leading obstetricians. He spoke to a rapt audience, and the next day's news referred to his method as "Readism" and "Readjustment." During his eleven-day visit he lectured at universities in Washington, Boston, Baltimore, and Chicago. At Yale he met Professor Thoms, who would be the first to introduce natural childbirth methods in an American teaching hospital. "It was more than I could have hoped for in my most ambitious moments," Dick-Read wrote afterward. "It was the first time I realized how fully many people outside my own country were waiting for this message."

Back in England, Dick-Read asked the Royal College of Obstetricians and Gynaecologists, still unsupportive of his ideas, for a hospital post in which he could teach his methods. They finally obliged, offering him a war-ravaged annex and no promise to repair the place.

Despondent over the lack of respect from his peers and a crumbling marriage, he accepted an invitation from a South African group that wanted to build a maternity hospital with Dick-Read at the helm. But when he arrived in Johannesburg, he once again faced resistance from the medical establishment. The South African Medical and Dental Council denied his registration to practice; he was forced to search elsewhere for work in the area. He found a small hospital run by Dominican nuns on the outskirts of the city, where he set up shop delivering babies using his all-natural method. There he filmed three births, offering the footage as proof to the world that his method worked.

Although Dick-Read continued to be shunned professionally, his ideas did catch on with the public, especially as women soured on hospital delivery practices. He died in 1959 and his hard-won fame was soon to be eclipsed by that of another obstetrician.

FERNAND LAMAZE

In 1910, lured by Paris and medical school, Fernand Lamaze abandoned life on a farm in the northeast of France. Within a few years, before settling on a professional specialty, he was pressed into army service during World War I. His time spent as an auxiliary physician removing bullets from thoraxes and watching bodies get nailed into white pine coffins ended abruptly when, on a summer day in 1917, a shell tore through his thigh. Lamaze married his field nurse. Back in Paris after the war ended, Lamaze's pregnant wife labored with their first child in their apartment. Upset by her anguished cries and his impotence to help, he left her in the bedroom with the obstetrician, headed for a bar, and drank a couple of bottles of wine. The next morning, wallowing in guilt and fear, he returned home to find a healthy daughter, a sleeping wife, and a tired doctor who lectured him on how obstetrics would be worthy of Lamaze's pursuit.

"Obstetrics never even crossed my mind," the doctor, nearing retirement, told Lamaze in hushed tones. "It was looked upon as a backwater profession. Women's labor was considered purely a physiologic function and without any fundamental connection to science. I took people's word for this, until one day I attended a frail, exhausted-looking woman who was going into labor. I had to perform the delivery alone. I had no experience. Medical school had only offered us theory. But I threw myself into what was one of the

most meaningful experiences of my life. Believe me, romantic inti-
macy pales in comparison to the bond an obstetrician feels with a
woman in labor. You become a creator. You are given the chance to
give life, to bring a human being out of the depths and into the light."

Those words, spoken in the quiet, somewhat shabby apartment where Lamaze's wife was lying-in, launched the career of a
man who would change the course of twentieth-century obstetrics.
Within ten years of his daughter's birth, Lamaze had become one
of the most respected obstetricians in Paris, no small feat in a city
that lays claim to inventing the field.

Yet Lamaze was a man of contradictions, catering to a bourgeois and upper-class clientele and practicing in a hospital run by
a metalworkers union. He told misogynist jokes, regularly cheated
on his wife with a mistress next door who ate dinners with his family, and frequented prostitutes. Despite all that, his career seemed
guided by a sense of humanity and respect for women. One night,
in 1924, Lamaze was called to a woman giving birth, one month
early, to a breech baby. The delivery dragged on for hours, ended
successfully, and moved him deeply. The next morning Lamaze
wrote in his diary: "[I] have finally lost my virginity."

Obstetrics became his obsession. The 1930s were busy for
obstetricians in France, a country intent on raising its birth rate.
The government literally was handing out medals to women after
they delivered.

In 1938, Lamaze first heard of Dick-Read's practice of "childbirth without fear." Lamaze agreed that fear caused—or at least
heightened—the awareness of pain. But Dick-Read's philosophy
of natural childbirth did not seem to grip the French obstetrician
as much as something he saw on a trip to the Soviet Union.

During World War II, Lamaze had harbored a communist
friend, Pierre Rouques, who later became the head of the metalworkers hospital. In 1951, too ill to travel with a French medical
delegation to the USSR, Rouques asked Lamaze to go in his place.

Lamaze accepted the invitation and found himself in Leningrad, watching a thirty-five-year-old woman give birth, in six hours, without anesthesia, to her first child. She was relaxed and showed no signs of pain.

"I had, at the time, thirty years of experience as an obstetrician. I had never been taught anything like this," Lamaze wrote in his classic 1956 book *Painless Childbirth: The Lamaze Method.* "I had never seen it; nor had I ever thought it could be possible. My emotional reaction was therefore all the stronger. I made a clean sweep of all preconceived ideas and, now an elderly schoolboy of sixty, I immediately decided to begin studying this new science."

The Soviet Union, where anesthesia was an unaffordable luxury, had adopted the theories of Ivan Petrovich Pavlov (1849–1936), a physiologist known for his famous experiments with dogs. Pavlov knew that when a dog saw food, it would begin salivating, a physiological reflex. In his experiments, he rang a bell when the food was placed in front of the dogs. Before long, the bell alone would cause the dogs' mouths to water, an act that is called a conditioned reflex. In another experiment, Pavlov applied an electric shock to a dog's paw. The dog, in a defensive reflex, barked and tried to get away as if in pain. Then Pavlov gave the dog a shock with food for several days. After a while, the defensive reflex weakened, until getting shocked merely caused the dog to salivate.

Pavlov applied these principles to laboring women, believing he could condition them to be desensitized to pain, just as he had the dogs. His method combined education about what to expect with breathing and relaxation techniques, including gently stroking the belly. Pavlov's method became the official system of obstetrical pain prevention in the USSR in 1951.

When Lamaze brought these ideas back from the Soviet Union, the western medical establishment believed the French doctor had been duped by the communist propaganda machine. But Lamaze was undeterred, and with Rouques's blessing, he transformed the metalworkers' clinic into the Maternité du Métal-lurgiste, a facility with fifty-two beds, enough for about two hundred deliveries every month. He had walls demolished to accommodate women for their birth preparation classes and trained everyone there—including the receptionist and the cleaning lady—in how to keep a mother relaxed. One crack in the birth-is-not-painful facade, he said, could ruin it for a mother-to-be.

Lamaze did not take the Pavlovian doctrine word for word, however. He replaced the deep breathing with huffing and puffing —he called this "the small dog" panting method—soon to become his hallmark. He believed such breathing was a diversion from the pain, as well as a way to oxygenate the blood, staving off exhaustion and breathlessness.

He also allowed pregnant women with abnormal fetus presentations such as breeches to participate in the training. Lamaze felt it was important to allow all women to use the method, even in a potentially more complicated birth such as a breech, because if a woman thought she was in a higher-risk situation, she would have even more trouble getting through it. Doubt, he believed—by the mother, her midwife, or a friend—was the greatest inhibitor to painless childbirth. In 1952, Madeleine Tsouladze became the first woman in France to give birth using the new Lamaze Method. Hers was a difficult breech birth but seemingly pain free. Publicity from the event made Lamaze so popular that women were registering at the small number of maternity hospitals that embraced the method, even before they became pregnant.

However, putting up a cheerful front that birth was not painful required a lot of work by a lot of people. Staff had to be retrained and pregnant women had to be educated. Several members of the hospital staff had to be by the mother's side throughout the entire labor and delivery—which for a first-time mother could last for days—to support her and keep her breathing focused. In the end, Lamaze could not overcome the government's concern about cost—and effectiveness. (Among the forty-five hundred women who delivered using his method at the Maternité du Métallurgiste over a 3½-year period, only 18 percent reported feeling no pain.)

The Lamaze Method, while popular in France, and later in the United States, never became a national orthodoxy the way the Pavlovian method, known as psychoprophylaxis, did in the USSR. For one thing, Lamaze annoyed the French medical establishment with his public campaign to have the government institute his method at a national level. He did this by showing the media a film of a Lamaze Method birth, during which the only cries came from the newborn; the movie made front-page headlines. The following year, in 1955, a recording of a Lamaze birth became a best-selling album. But the Medical Board called him in for "false advertising," and the clinic began to rescind its funding of his efforts.

On March 5, 1957, the metalworkers held a stormy meeting with Lamaze, essentially putting an end to his great experiment. The next morning, he died.

Psychoprophylaxis—it was still not yet called the "Lamaze Method"—had begun to spread among women in Europe and America. The timing, at the peak of the Cold War, made western doctors uneasy, and they openly questioned whether it was politically correct for them to allow women to try something that had originated behind the Iron Curtain. In addition, old-school Catholic obstetricians wanted to know whether the technique was religiously acceptable. In 1956, about seven hundred doctors from around the world gathered for a gynecological symposium with Pope Pius XII at the Vatican, which still opposed the use of pain-relief drugs for childbirth.

"How do you feel about the Russian method of painless childbirth?" one attendee asked the pope, who was seated on his throne. The pope, speaking in French, said that although the method had originated in an atheistic culture, he found nothing immoral about it.

"There are some who allege that originally childbirth was entirely painless and that it became painful only at a later date (perhaps due to an erroneous interpretation of the judgment of God) as a result of autosuggestion and heterosuggestion, arbitrary associations, conditioned reflexes, and because of faulty behavior of mothers in labor," the pope said. "Science and technique can, therefore, use the conclusions of experimental psychology, of physiology and of gynecology (as in the psycho-prophylactic method) . . . to render childbirth as painless as possible."

Catholics and communist-haters, women and doctors alike, who wanted births without guilt or drugs, were delighted to have the pope's consent.

Meanwhile, Marjorie Karmel, the American who had sought out Lamaze while she was living in Paris, had moved to New York and published her book *Thank You, Dr. Lamaze,* exporting his ideas to the world's English-speaking population. The book was a revelation to many women who believed shackles, enemas, and anesthesia should no longer be routine in U.S. maternity wards.

Another New York mother, Elisabeth Bing, was so moved by Karmel's book that she called the author, then living on the other side of Central Park. They met, became friends, and together established the American Society for Psychoprophylaxis in Obstetrics, or ASPO, in 1960. The group launched the era of childbirth classes in the United States after Bing imported a film called *Naissance,* showing a drug-free labor and delivery with typical French anatomical candor.

"It was very important to show it to the public, not just the nurses," Bing said recently in her sunny Upper West Side apartment, above the space where she gave childbirth classes for decades. "We ran into difficulty. The hospital or the YWCA or whatever organization wouldn't show it. They thought it was pornographic."

They screened the film for couples in Karmel's larger Upper East Side apartment. The media began reporting on the classes, and soon the public demanded access to childbirth education. Though Karmel died of cancer in 1964, Bing continued to give the Lamaze Method classes. In 1970, only 10 percent of U.S. hospitals sponsored prenatal courses. By 1975, most did.

"It was a consumer movement," Bing said. "It wasn't really a movement by Lamaze or Read or me. The time was ripe. It was a time when the public doubted everything their parents had done."

Bing, now in her nineties, taught her last class in 2004, on the first floor of the building where she lives. The space, featuring maroon carpeting, warm and dark like a womb, had recently been emptied of everything but some art. One wall had a collection of pre-Columbian birthing statues. Another wall had vintage depictions of the baby in utero at different stages of birth. There were two large

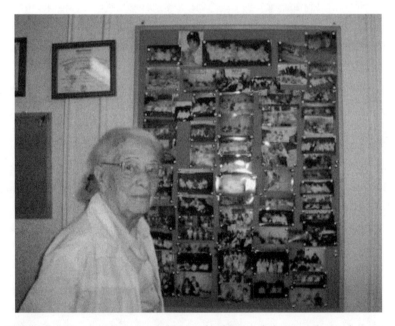

Elisabeth Bing, standing near photos of babies and their mothers who graduated from her Upper West Side birthing classes, held in the room where she was photographed in 2005. (Photo by Tina Cassidy)

bulletin boards filled with baby snapshots her graduates had sent. And then there was the cartoon poster showing a female construction worker nursing a child, homage to how popular natural childbirth had become. The cartoon, taped to the door, was curling at the edges.

By 1997, the American Society for Psychoprophylaxis in Obstetrics had become Lamaze International, a nonprofit group that today has three thousand certified educators working across thirty-two countries, from Korea to Kenya, teaching women not that birth is pain free, but that the pain is manageable.

While Lamaze's technique of educating women about the physiologic process of birth continues in a major way, little else of the French doctor's original method remains in common practice. For one thing, most birth instructors today will tell you not to pant. It can cause hyperventilation.

So what is the legacy of Lamaze? The classes now emphasize that birth is normal and it's best to get through it without drugs or technological interference. The group also promotes breast-feeding and publishes *Lamaze Magazine,* which refuses to accept advertisements from baby formula companies despite the financial windfall that would result from doing so. Instead, as a way of generating revenue, Lamaze has licensed its name to the Learning Curve toy company, which sells twenty-four-inch velour inchworms that rattle, crinkle, and play "If you're happy and you know it, clap your hands" for $14.99.

EMANUEL FRIEDMAN

While Fernand Lamaze remains widely known, Dr. Emanuel Friedman is recognized by few outside the medical community. Yet his obstetrical contribution, devised around the same time that Lamaze rose to fame, still changes birth outcomes every day, all over the world.

In the late 1940s, on the recommendation of a professor, Friedman ditched math and science for obstetrics. But his earlier interests would not be wasted. As a medical student at Columbia University, Friedman walked into a labor room and saw Dr. Virginia Apgar (for whom Apgar scores are named) explaining the virtues of caudal anesthesia, a precursor to the epidural. "She took my finger and my thumb and placed it on her caudal notch," said Friedman, bemused by the memory of having to touch Apgar's backside. "I think I was far more embarrassed than educated." A couple of years later, as an OB resident at Columbia-Presbyterian's Sloane Hospital for Women in New York, he was looking for a project, and Apgar suggested that, given his math background, he look into what caudal anesthesia did to the process of labor. Did it slow? Did it speed up? Recalled Friedman, "The prime objective was [to determine] what the impact of anesthesia was on the course of labor."

At the time, residents were not supposed to be married; all their time and attention was to be devoted in priestly fashion to their work. Friedman was not only married—something he did not publicize—but his wife was pregnant with their first child. On June 10, 1951, she went into labor. He was not allowed to leave the hospital to be with her. Distraught, he put his nervous energy to use during the busy overnight shift in his own obstetrics ward. With Apgar's suggestion in mind, he checked in on all twenty-five women at regular intervals throughout their labor, regardless of whether they had anesthesia.

"I was plotting out all the things I could possibly examine for on a simple graph," Friedman recalled. "It was clear by morning that dilation of the cervix and descent of the fetus were easily recognizable mathematical processes."

When the sun came up, the Friedmans' first child, a girl, had not yet entered the world. That would happen later in the day. But Friedman's "cervimetric curve" had been born. This was a bell-shaped graph that tracked what no one had tracked before: the av-

erage length of time of the three stages of labor. His simple averages would help doctors determine if their patient's progress was
well outside the norm. Friedman found that in the latent phase of
the first stage of labor, when contractions tend to be neither regular nor painful, the woman can dilate as much as four centimeters
over an average of 8.6 hours, although first-time mothers might take
much longer. However—and this was significant—Friedman's
curve emphasized that active labor, the period when contractions
become regular, strong, and painful, was the true measure of
whether labor is progressing normally. At the time, many doctors
believed in the folk wisdom that the sun shall not set twice on a
woman in labor. If doctors were monitoring the latent phase of the
first stage of labor and found it to be taking too long, the woman
could be subjected to an unnecessary cesarean or other intervention long before her body was truly working to expel the baby.

Friedman also determined that during active labor, dilation
to eight centimeters takes an average of 2.5 hours, with the cervix
opening more slowly until it is fully dilated at 10 centimeters. The
second stage of labor, when the woman pushes, takes an average
of 1 hour for first babies and 15 minutes for later births. (The third
stage is the expulsion of the placenta.)

The frustration for Friedman, an emeritus professor at
Harvard, is that doctors have used his averages, first published in
1954, as rigid benchmarks for monitoring labor's progress, without considering how many women fall on either side of his
asymmetrical bell curve. There is a wide range of "normal," Friedman says, admitting he's distressed and disappointed by how the
curve is misused to diagnose a woman's failure to progress, the
most common reason American doctors list on charts for justify-
ing a C-section.

This is not how it was supposed to be. He had intended the
curve to be a simple visual tool to help obstetricians, midwives, and
patients determine if and when labor might be deviating widely—

his carefully chosen words—from the normal range. Before he plotted the curve, there was no standard for normal.

"We found an average. People think the average is what women should fall upon. That is clearly not true but rather a broad range of normality beyond which a potential abnormality may or may not exist. Those abnormalities are not in themselves justification for forceps or cesarean. . . . It doesn't mean she's doing so badly that you have to do something terrible to her. That is being abused."

VIRGINIA APGAR

Virginia Apgar, the woman who cheekily embarrassed Friedman at the start of his medical career, suspected hospitals might be abusing something else: obstetric anesthesia. This was a startling accusation given Apgar's standing. She was a woman physician at a time when medicine was dominated by men, and she was an anesthesiologist.

Yet Apgar was determined and self-assured. She had excelled in medical school during the Great Depression, graduating fourth in her class despite the added pressure of financial hardship. Although she had won a surgical internship through Columbia University, the chief surgeon there persuaded her to switch fields, directing her toward anesthesiology, a lower-paying field that, at the time, was not considered a true medical specialty. After training in Wisconsin, she returned to Columbia to run the anesthesiology department. Few physicians, however, wanted to work for her, which probably had as much to do with her being a woman as with the fact that there was little prestige surrounding anesthesiology. Apgar, however, knew that the field held promise, and she began investigating obstetrical anesthesia, which was pervasive at the time.

Finding that babies delivered by anesthetized mothers needed special attention in the critical minutes after birth, she devised a simple test to evaluate the condition of the baby's heart rate, respiration, reflex irritability, muscle tone, and color. Sixty seconds after the complete birth of the baby, a rating of 0, 1, or 2 points was given in each of the five categories, depending on whether the condition was absent or present. A perfect score was 10.

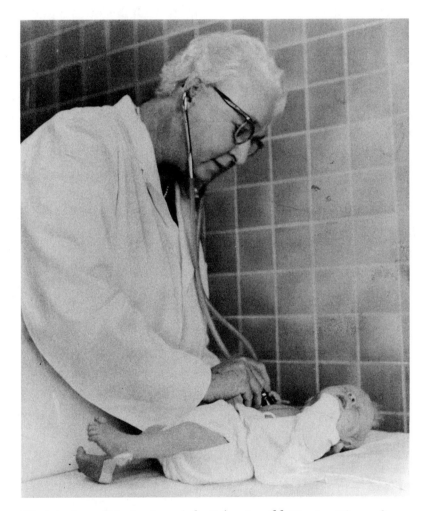

Virginia Apgar listening to an infant's heart, 1966 (Courtesy Library of Congress, Prints and Photographs Division, New York World)

In 1953, after rating more than a thousand newborns at the hospital, Apgar found that babies in the best condition were natural (not anesthetized) vaginal deliveries, with an average score of 8.4, followed by cesarean births at 8 points when the mother had a spinal, and 5 points when she was under general anesthesia. Breeches averaged 6.3 points. Apgar also correlated the scores with death rates and found that the newborns with the lowest figures were the most likely to perish.

Apgar's test, which earned her an honorary U.S. postage stamp, is even more remarkable because her method has endured in a profession that is constantly evolving. Consider: J. Marion Sims closed holes; Joseph B. DeLee made them bigger. Grantly Dick-Read believed that birth was a simple physiological process; Fernand Lamaze believed that, with a little practice, labor and delivery could be controlled by the mind. Emanuel Friedman used numbers to help women through labor; Apgar used numbers to save babies, by directing resources to those with perilously low scores. Of course, Apgar is the only doctor included here who was not an obstetrician. But that's not surprising given that, throughout history, obstetrics has been the realm of men. Which begs the question: Would the profession have been gentler on women or babies if it were not overrun with men and their tools? Perhaps not. Today, the majority of new OBs in America are female, and with intervention rates higher than ever, it's clear that women can order a Pitocin drip, perform a C-section, and maneuver a vacuum extractor as good as the next guy.

7 TOOLS AND FADS

GIVING BIRTH CAN make a perfectly dignified woman walk naked in front of strangers, threaten to murder her husband, or tell a nurse to stuff it. Women have tolerated unnatural labor positions, "little snips," humiliating enemas, unnecessary shavings, dangerous instruments, embarrassing hospital gowns, and tight labor schedules for hundreds of years. They've been told to pant like dogs, deliver under water, bounce on balls, let doulas draw pretty pictures on their backs, listen to classical music, and burn scented candles. They've been primed to ask for that year's drug of choice.

Twilight Sleep is in. Twilight Sleep is out. Forceps are in. Forceps are out. Episiotomies are in. Episiotomies are out. What is state of the art one year is outmoded and unfathomable the next, leaving us to laugh at the hocus pocus, marvel at how mothers are thrilled by some new "easy" way, or recoil in horror at the damage done. In Colonial America, doctors believed drawing blood from a laboring woman could relieve pain, stop convulsions in those with puerperal fever, accelerate labor, soften a rigid cervix, and help ease the birth of a baby coming feet first. Physicians even bled women who were hemorrhaging, believing that reducing circulation further would make the blood clot. The woman might faint from the blood loss; in this new, relaxed state, her body could open up enough to make way for the baby. But sometimes there

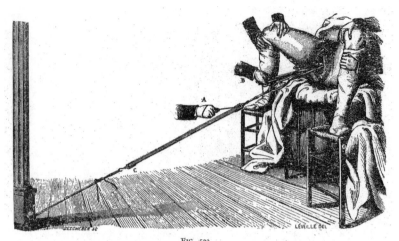

FIG. 522.
Delore's method of mechanical traction by means of pulleys and cords.

*This image, published in Calcutta in 1929, shows a gruesome method of
pulling with forceps. (Courtesy the Wellcome Library)*

were deadly consequences. The wife of Salmon P. Chase, Abraham
Lincoln's secretary of the treasury, spiked a fever after her delivery. Hoping to bring down her temperature, doctors withdrew fifty
ounces of blood. Her pulse, and her strength, steadily weakened.
Then she died.

Some of the more remarkable obstetric fads were not methods or techniques at all. They were tools. And their vast permuta-
tions over the centuries tell dramatic stories of difficult births, of
ignorant attempts to help, and of swashbuckling stupidity. As part
of my research for this book, I visited the College of Physicians of
Philadelphia's Mütter Museum, a dignified if macabre facility, devoted to the history of medicine. Their obstetrical instrument collection is so huge that the vast majority of the forceps, cranium
perforators, fetal decapitators, symphysis knives, hooks, and fistula repair kits have to be stored in metal cabinet drawers in the
museum's cramped basement. The storeroom is down the stairs
from the displays of antique bone specimens, which include pel-

vises deformed by rickets and rib cages malformed by corsets—
both of which serve as reminders of why many of these tools were
invented in the first place.

The drawers—packed with such horrifying gadgets as spiral
"curettes" for removing placentas; pessaries; and dozens of forceps
spanning hundreds of years—also contained some of the simplest
obstetric tools ever made: levers, blunt hooks, and *crochets.*

The lever, which looks like a cross between a long shoe horn
and a crow bar, was used in the 1600s to try to dislodge stuck fetuses. By the 1740s, the lever was replaced with a vectis, similar
to its predecessor except that the spoon end had an oval cut out of
it. This fenestrated tool was essentially one half a pair of forceps,
which only recently had made its public debut. Another early tool
was the L-shaped blunt hook, which featured a long arm with a
wooden handle. Attendants would use it to put pressure on the
fetus's body (but not destroy it). Surgeons commonly used the
blunt hook in breech cases.

The *crochet,* a French term for a small hook, was a far more
devastating tool. Angled with a sharp V on one end and a softer
curve on the other, the tool would have been used in craniotomy
cases to remove brain tissue and apply traction to body parts. The
crochet was equally dangerous for the mother, whose birth canal
was easily perforated by it. A report in 1829 said half of the mothers whose pregnancies ended with a craniotomy died themselves.
One solution was to envelop the hook in tubes, which protected
the mother as the fetus was being extracted.

Tools did not necessarily become safer with time, although
they did become more elaborate. One can see a neat progression
of how the instruments were increasingly designed to make the
surgeon's job easier. A French physician named Baudeloque
replaced the *crochet* with a *cephalotribe,* all two feet and seven
pounds of it. The device had two enormous blades that could crush
a fetal skull with a twist of a hand crank before compressing the

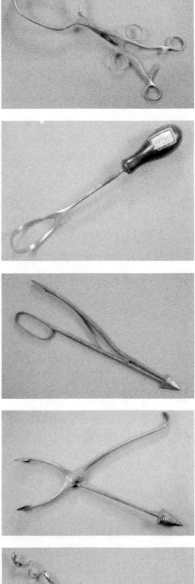

Undated basiotribe, used for crushing the fetal skull. *(Courtesy the Mütter Museum)*

Undated vectis, used to gain traction on fetal head. *(Courtesy the Mütter Museum)*

Undated fetal skull perforator. *(Courtesy the Mütter Museum)*

Undated combination tool for piercing, crushing, and removing fetal head. *(Courtesy the Mütter Museum)*

An undated "curette" for removing the placenta. *(Courtesy the Mütter Museum)*

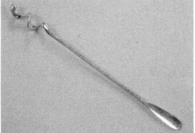

head and pulling it out. A less complicated version of that tool was called a *basiotribe*.

While it was fascinating to inspect each of these crude tools, I had really hoped to find a set of Chamberlen forceps, the grand-daddy of obstetric tools. The legend behind the Chamberlen forceps, named after the barber-surgeon who, in the 1500s, designed the first useful set of "iron hands," is as intriguing as the tool itself.

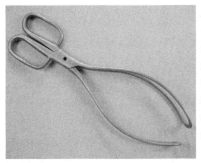

A seventeenth-century version of Chamberlen-style forceps, which would have been united with a removable screw or braided cord passed through the small hole between the joint and tied with a knot at one end, allowing the operator to bring together or disunite the blades when needed. (Courtesy the Mütter Museum)

Although other cultures and midwives may have used forceps-like devices much earlier—the Japanese used whale bones the way we use forceps today—Peter Chamberlen's rudimentary forceps, designed in the late sixteenth century, were meant to remove a baby without necessarily destroying it. The fenestrated blades were short and straight, with slightly rounded edges. The handles were similar to those on scissors but more awkward to hold; the attendant would have had to skillfully place a blade on each side of the fetal head without causing damage or repeated slippage and then try to fasten the two blades back together before pulling.

Chamberlen, born in Paris in 1560, lived in England and learned some midwifery from his sister. He did not let mothers he attended see his closely guarded tools, which he kept locked in a huge wooden box adorned with gilt carvings. The box was so heavy that when Chamberlen was called to a birth, it took two men to carry it to the lying-in chamber, the door of which he'd lock behind him to keep out any witnesses.

Five generations of Chamberlen men guarded the secret instruments. Women and midwives would pay them a huge fee, about ten thousand dollars in today's market, to help retrieve a stuck baby. The Chamberlens were zealous about keeping their invention out of the hands of their competitors, even if their greed imperiled women and babies. The family was regularly in trouble with the authorities, whether it was for prescribing drugs to patients—something barber-surgeons were not allowed to do—or for not paying debts, which landed Peter, the inventor, temporarily behind bars.

His descendants carried on the family practice by soliciting—actually, that may be too kind a word—business from midwives by hosting elaborate dinners for them or offering to build alms houses. Eventually, one descendant, Hugh Chamberlen, decided he could profit more by selling the tools to others than by keeping them a secret. In 1673, he traveled to Paris to meet France's preeminent *accoucheur*, François Mauriceau, at the Hotel Dieu. Mauriceau pioneered the stitching of torn perineums (after cleansing them with red wine) and delivering breeches by inserting a finger in the baby's mouth. He, too, perpetuated the practice of delivering women on their backs in bed.

Although Mauriceau already had his own set of destructive implements, including the frightfully named *tire-tête,* or "head puller," Chamberlen hoped the Frenchman would be willing to pay a huge sum for the set of secret forceps that he believed could deliver anyone.

Mauriceau was skeptical. He tested Chamberlen's device in his delivery of a twenty-eight-year-old pregnant woman whose pelvis was warped by rickets and whose water had broken four days earlier. Mauriceau believed a most certainly lethal cesarean was the only option—unless Chamberlen actually had something worth buying. Chamberlen jumped at the chance to demonstrate and applied the forceps to the fetal head. But after three hours of ceaseless effort, he failed to extract the child. The mother died the next day when Mauriceau performed a cesarean, too late. Her uterus had ruptured; the fetus was dead.

Chamberlen returned to England and spent the next ten years working on a land bank stock scheme, which also failed. He then turned his attention back to forceps, traveling to Holland, where, in 1693, he allegedly sold his instrument to a surgeon, who then shared the concept with the Medico-Pharmaceutical College of Amsterdam, which granted the rights to others to use them. Trouble was, Chamberlen—or the local surgeon, it is not clear who perpetrated the fraud—offered only a single blade to the college. (They did not know there should be two blades!) The concept, however, was enough to set other inventors in motion.

Given all the secrecy surrounding the original Chamberlen design, how do we know what the tools really looked like? After Hugh Chamberlen died in 1683, it appears that his wife placed his original forceps in a box, and stored them beneath a trap door in the floorboards of a closet in their English home. There the forceps stayed for one hundred and thirty years. In 1813, new owners of the house discovered the box, filled with several pairs of short, straight forceps that eventually were turned over to the Royal Medical and Chirurgical Society.

By the mid-1700s, others had already begun to improve upon the Chamberlen design. Smellie added the pelvic curve—a

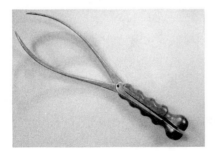

Eighteenth-century Smellie-style forceps, with finger grips on handles and blades bent to fit shape of the birth canal.
(Courtesy the Mütter Museum)

bend in the blade to conform to the shape of the woman's birth canal. Over time, forceps blades became longer, allowing barber-surgeons to reach for the baby before the head had even entered the pelvis. Attendants believed they were doing the mother a favor by going in after the baby earlier in labor and saving her from the pain of contractions.

"I take pride in stating that, as far as my recollection goes, in no case of my own was a woman ever allowed to lie in suffering and danger till the os [cervix] was 'completely dilated,'" one doctor wrote in the *Journal of the American Medical Association* in the mid-1880s, when the debate about when to use forceps was still raging. Of course, extracting the baby that soon—before full dilation—was dangerous, even deadly. The tongs could grip the womb as well as the head; in such cases, when the doctor yanked, the baby would be delivered along with shreds of uterine tissue or the placenta, causing potentially fatal hemorrhage.

Physicians used forceps more and more during the Industrial Revolution, when rickets became pervasive. Women increasingly understood that the tools could ease a difficult birth, possibly saving the fetus from a craniotomy. Eventually, the hands of steel became a sign of prestige, and women expected doctors to use them regardless of need. They were not always the life-savers many hoped them to be, however. In the hands of unskilled operators, the tools lacerated the mother, introduced infection, and damaged babies' brains, eyes, ears, noses, and facial nerves.

Dan Millikin, a nineteenth-century doctor in Hamilton, Ohio, candidly wrote in a medical journal about trying to deliver a baby with forceps before the head was fully engaged in the pelvis. He soon realized that the child was coming out feet first, and when he inserted the forceps, one blade got stuck. "Then my hand, passed into the uterus, revealed the fact that the child's right hand had passed through the fenestrum of the [forceps] and that, in fact, the blade hung on the bend of the elbow, as a basket hangs on one's arm. . . . Presently, when the child had been delivered by the feet, it was seen that violence had been done to the forearm."

Some forceps were intentionally destructive. James Young Simpson devised the craniotomy forceps to replace the cephalotribe around 1870. A surgeon would insert one blade in the already perforated skull, while the other blade crushed the head. A more advanced type of craniotomy forceps had spikes on one blade and convex holes in the other, to simultaneously perforate and remove the fetal skull.

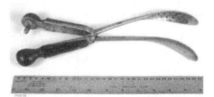

Craniotomy forceps. (Courtesy the Mütter Museum)

At the beginning of the twentieth century, about half of all American deliveries were by forceps. In more modern times, doctors stopped using high forceps—for use when the cervix was not fully dilated. Instead, they used mid-range forceps when the baby's head was engaged in the pelvis but was not on the pelvic floor; or low-range forceps when the baby's head was on the pelvic floor. In the early twentieth century, nearly half of all American births still involved forceps, but by 1994 they were used less than 4 percent of the time. Other methods to help difficult deliveries were encroaching—specifically, cesarean sections and vacuums.

THE VACUUM

The idea of the vacuum originated in ancient times, when medical practitioners heated a metal cup over a flame and placed it on a wound; as the cup cooled, it created a vacuum that suctioned out blood and other fluids. In the sixteenth century, Ambroise Paré— the French surgeon who instructed women to deliver lying down— discovered that he could correct compressed fractures in an infant's skull by applying a leather "sucker," which was essentially a slab of wet leather with a string attached to the center. The leather formed an airtight seal which was then yanked to pull out the dent. Others experimented with this idea using fish bladders instead of leather.

In 1836, James Young Simpson saw a group of boys playing "suckers," a competition to see who could lift the largest stone using wet leather threaded to a string. This chance encounter, and perhaps some knowledge of Paré's work, pushed Simpson to devise a prototype vacuum to extract a fetus. Such a device would require more powerful suction than a slab of leather could provide, and Simpson began researching other materials. Within a few years, he had perfected his invention, and he presented his rubber "*ventouse*" to a large crowd at the Medical Chirurgical Society. He demonstrated by fixing the suction to the palm of his right hand and lifting a twenty-eight-pound weight attached to it. Still, some physicians doubted that the device could work well in practice. So Simpson took them to view a "baddish case and fixed the tractor on. The operation was most successful," he later wrote. His early design involved a leather-covered metal speculum with a piston fitted inside to pull out the air and create a vacuum. He greased with lard the end that attached to the head and "sucked" out the baby. His first practical "air tractor" hit the market in 1849.

Over the next hundred years, many physicians invented their own vacuum designs, altering the shape of the cup as well as the process for suction, which included using foot and hand pumps. But it was not until Tage Malmström of Sweden created a stainless-steel cup device in the 1950s that the vacuum extractor's prospects grew. However, ongoing problems with product design and serious fetal complications continued to stifle obstetricians'

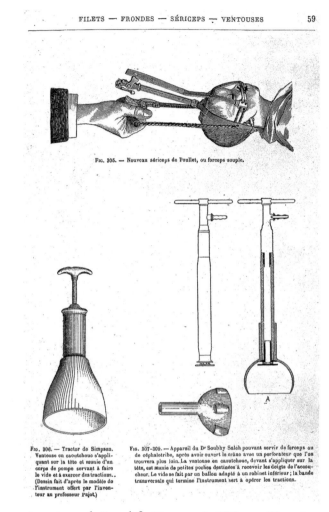

FIG. 305. — Nouveau sériceps de Poullet, ou forceps souple.

FIG. 306. — Tractor de Simpson. Ventouse en caoutchouc s'appliquant sur la tête et munie d'un corps de pompe servant à faire le vide et à exercer des tractions. (Dessin fait d'après le modèle de l'instrument offert par l'inventeur au professeur Pajot.)

FIG. 307-309. — Appareil du Dr Soubhy Saleh pouvant servir de forceps ou de céphalotribe, après avoir ouvert le crâne avec un perforateur que l'on trouvera plus loin. La ventouse en caoutchouc, devant s'appliquer sur la tête, est munie de petites poches destinées à recevoir les doigts de l'accoucheur. Le vide se fait par un ballon adapté à un robinet inférieur ; la bande transversale qui termine l'instrument sert à opérer les tractions.

Simpson's ventouse, bottom left. (Courtesy the Wellcome Library)

interest. The vacuum did not come truly into vogue until the 1980s, when widespread epidural use diminished the ability of women to successfully push.

Modern obstetricians, especially the younger ones, favor vacuums—which have benefited from improved designs—over forceps because they result in fewer maternal injuries, such as trauma to the anal sphincter, or the need for an episiotomy to make room for the forceps. The vacuum is also less likely to damage the fetus because the suction is applied to the bony top of the head, although it does cause the newborn to enter the world with its cranium shaped like a hair bun. (Actually, doctors refer to this molding effect as a chignon.)

Using a vacuum is a delicate science, however. The position of the baby's head must be carefully considered. If the cup will not attach easily to the head, doctors quickly will abandon their efforts in favor of a cesarean because, most likely, the head and pelvis are disproportionate or the head is in a bad position. About fifty thousand American babies are born with the help of a vacuum every year, 85 percent of them delivered with four or fewer pulls on the extractor.

ULTRASOUND

Forceps and vacuums, despite their evolution, are decidedly low tech compared with a new technology that could see inside the womb.

In 1906, American Lewis Nixon invented a sound-wave device to detect icebergs. Fascinating technology, to be sure, but no one really thought to use it until the *Titanic* sank in 1912. Around the same time, the American military, perhaps foreseeing World War I and eventual underwater naval battles, began to develop the technology to hunt submarines. By 1914, the first working sonar system in the United States was up and running, capable of also spotting icebergs underwater two miles away.

Soon after, Frenchman Paul Langevin discovered that high-intensity ultrasound could destroy schools of fish in the ocean, and when a person put a hand in a tank of water that had ultrasound waves running through it, they experienced pain, a discovery that led doctors to use the technology to destroy tissue, such as a brain tumor.

Doctors in the 1940s hailed the technology as a cure-all for everything from eczema to arthritis. By World War II, Americans were calling the technology sonar—an acronym for sound, navigation, and ranging—hence the term sonogram. It was as good for spotting gallstones, breast tumors, and rectal obstructions as for finding U-boats.

In the late 1950s, doctors began adapting the technology to help them see into another watery world: the uterus. Scotsman Ian Donald, a World War I veteran and gadget junkie, had been using sonar experimentally in his ob-gyn work. In 1958, he published a groundbreaking article in *Lancet* describing how he had found a large ovarian cyst using the sonar technology. By 1959, the bulky ultrasound machine could produce clear echoes of the shape of a baby *in utero* and could diagnose multiple pregnancies and placenta previa.

At first, doctors required pregnant women to be in a bath to have an ultrasound; they later realized water-soluble jelly could more easily transmit the ultrasound waves. Today, the machines are nimble, handheld devices that generate clear, real-time pictures showing everything from fetal heart deformities to whether the baby is already sucking his or her thumb.

Technicians routinely perform ultrasounds around the fourth month of pregnancy in order to spot fetal abnormalities and estimate a due date; as a bonus, many parents get to glimpse the gender of the child or see the profile of its nose. But the free market has taken ultrasound one step further. In the last few years, companies with names such as Stork Snapshots and First Glimpse have begun offering ultrasound "portraits"—amber-hued, high-definition, three-dimensional fetal images suitable for framing or DVD viewing.

Critics of the technology, however, are concerned that the scans can cause unknown problems.

"We do know that in the short term cells behave abnormally after just one diagnostic ultrasound exposure," writes Susan

McCutcheon, author of *Natural Childbirth the Bradley Way.* "The shape of cells so radiated changes temporarily and their movement becomes frenetic."

Sheila Kitzinger, a British author and childbirth expert, also stresses caution when it comes to using an ultrasound. "As far as we know, ultrasound is safe, certainly much safer than X-rays," Kitzinger writes. "On the other hand, it is known that high frequency sound waves continued for a long time can damage an adult's hearing. Questions have therefore been raised about effects on the baby's hearing, since, although the sound waves are bounced off the baby for only a short time, the baby may be vulnerable at certain stages of its development. Babies are not born deaf after having ultrasound in the uterus, but no one yet knows if any of them will suffer delayed effects later in life."

The U.S. Food and Drug Administration states that women should avoid unnecessary ultrasound and that the 3-D pictures are an unapproved use of a medical device. But parents don't seem to be worried. In fact, many of the services allow moms and dads to come back a second time free of charge if the fetus did not reveal its gender on the first visit. A $295 "platinum" package at one franchise allows parents to come back in the last trimester just to see how much the baby has grown and get a better view of its facial features.

This mounting anticipation at the end of pregnancy, combined with increasing physical discomfort and the desire to control the timing of the delivery, is spawning a new phenomenon. Many women are begging to be induced—and their obstetricians are complying.

INDUCTION

Labor induction is an ancient practice typically performed because the fetus was dead or the mother was ill. In the last several hundred years, midwives began more commonly inducing labor in pregnant women who had rickets, hoping a younger, and therefore smaller, fetus would be more able to fit through the pelvis. In the twentieth century, obstetricians were likely to induce labor if the mother had severely high blood pressure, a condition known as preeclampsia, or simply because she was past her due date, the baby getting larger by the hour.

Different cultures have had their own techniques for starting—and augmenting—labor, from shaking the woman on a blanket to suspending her from a tree, or giving her sneezing powders such as red pepper, blown through a goose quill up the nose. In the Yucatán, midwives offered raw egg to a laboring woman to make her gag, an act that could bring on stronger contractions probably because vomiting releases oxytocin. Nipple stimulation (recommended even in ancient times, by Hippocrates), intercourse, hot baths, and vigorous leg massages also can crank up a woman's labor.

The Hopi of North America fed weasels to pregnant women because the swift animal is known for working its way through the ground and finding a way out. Another Native American tribe, the Paiute, believed that if the woman reduced the amount she ate near the end of the pregnancy the fetus would slowly starve and try to leave the womb. As a bonus, they believed that through fasting, the woman's birth canal would become less thick, allowing the child to pass more easily. The Jivaro headhunters of the Amazon also fed the woman eggs, thinking that she would make like a hen and lay one herself. The Maori of New Zealand played a phallus-shaped flute made from ancestral bones whose spirits might assist her in getting the baby out. And in the Auvergne region of France, midwives plopped a chicken on the woman's belly, theorizing that its scratchy feet would begin or accelerate labor.

Some cultures used scare tactics. The Siwa of Egypt would fire two rifles near the woman to speed up labor. In ancient times, midwives might thump on the pregnant woman's belly, hoping to make the baby flee its comfortable spot. Native Americans were said to charge the would-be mother with a horse, pulling away at the last minute in an effort to frighten the child into the world. The Germans also believed that scaring the mother could accelerate a protracted labor and sometimes flogged pregnant women in an attempt to frighten and bring forth the baby. Royalty, of course, could not be flogged, and in the case of one German empress with a stalled labor, attendants brought twenty-four men, one after the other, into her chamber so *they* could be whacked. Two of the men died. The violence didn't help much. The labor inched along at a snail's pace.

A more effective induction method was to give a woman the fungus called ergot. Ergot has the ability to cause powerful contractions. Used since ancient times, it had to be administered with care because a high dosage could cause massive contractions leading to uterine rupture. If it was ingested after the placenta was expelled, however, the strong contractions could prevent fatal hemorrhage, and ergot certainly was useful for reactivating a stalled labor, especially from a doctor's perspective.

"It expedites lingering parturition, and saves to the *accoucheur* a considerable portion of time, without producing any bad effects on the patient," wrote John Stearns, a New York doctor who is credited with making the fungus's application more mainstream in the early 1800s. Stearns's technique involved gathering ergot from a granary where rye was stored. He recommended putting some of the powdered fungus in a pint of boiling water, which the woman, mostly dilated already, would drink in thirds every twenty minutes until contractions began. Otherwise, he gave her five to ten grains of powdered ergot. But generally, Stearns found the effects to be so quick that he warned other physicians to be prepared for the birth before administering ergot. "Since I have adopted the use of this powder I have seldom found a case detained me more than three hours," Stearns boasted.

In the 1800s, there were few other options for inducing labor, none of them great: Rupturing the membranes could lead to infection; bloodletting could deplete a woman's blood supply to the point that she fainted or died; and streaming tepid water into the vagina to separate the membranes from the uterine wall often led to uterine rupture and very high maternal mortality. In the mid-1800s, some attendants inserted sponges into the vagina to stimulate dilation. In 1891, a published study of one hundred early-induction cases showed how some of the above methods had lethal consequences, leading to the death of one mother and thirty-three newborns. But physicians weren't sure what else to do with an inactive uterus. In the early 1900s, DeLee used balloons to dilate cervixes. (Doctors still do this.)

Because such methods often caused infection, doctors tried other, less invasive remedies, including administering doses of castor oil, which caused the woman to gag or vomit. Throughout the 1920s, doctors also experimented with taking extract from the pituitary gland and placing it in the nostril of the patient to stimulate the uterus. This turned out to be dangerous—infant death in these cases exceeded 6 percent.

In the years after 1949, pharmaceutical advancements led to the development of synthetic oxytocin, commonly known as Pitocin, which was easily administered through an intravenous line. Its use skyrocketed. By 1978, Britain had a 40 percent induction rate, three times what it was in 1958. As many as 75 percent of the patients of certain physicians were being induced, a trend that reflected the growing desire—by doctors—to manage deliveries so that births occurred during business hours.

Between 1970 and 1976, British births were most likely to happen between Monday and Friday, with Sunday being the least likely day for a delivery. "Relatively few births occurred on bank holidays, especially Christmas Day and Boxing Day," according to a 1978 report in the *British Medical Journal*. Obstetricians said the

177

trend had improved their job satisfaction and made the running of maternity departments easier.

"In some hospitals it was surmised that the quality of obstetric care was better in the day-time than at night," said another report that same year. "From this it was a short step to consider that the care provided might also be better on weekdays than at weekends when facilities were likely to be less adequately staffed."

In the United States, induction rates more than doubled between 1989 and 1998, from 10 percent to 20 percent. But many believe the rate is grossly underestimated. In a 2002 survey, nearly half of the women asked said they had been artificially induced.

The reasons for caution are many. An induced labor is riskier than one that begins on its own. Not only is it more painful—Pitocin causes fierce contractions—induction is more likely to lead to fetal distress, more likely to require pain relief, more likely to end in cesarean, and more likely to cause a previous uterine scar to rupture. Some parents and researchers have even suggested that there is a link between the Pitocin epidemic and the higher incidence of autism since the mid-1980s.

Doctors are likely to induce mothers who are past their forty-week "due date" out of concern that the baby might get too big for an uncomplicated delivery. But statistics show that half of all healthy first-time mothers have pregnancies that last longer than forty-one weeks, and their births are fine.

ENEMAS

There's one other method that has been used for centuries to bring on labor: The enema. Forcing warm water into a pregnant woman's rectum was an ancient tradition unfortunately slow to die, first promulgated by midwives who believed in its induction powers, then by physicians who thought childbed fever was spread through accidental bowel movements during the pushing phase.

"In 1900 each patient at Sloane [maternity hospital in New York] received an enema immediately upon admission and then a vaginal douche with biochloride of mercury, the favored antiseptic. Nurses then washed the woman's head with kerosene, ether, and ammonia, her nipples and umbilicus with ether; they shaved the pubic hair of charity patients, assuming that poor people harbored more germs, and clipped it for private patients. They gave a woman in labor an enema every 12 hours and continued to douche the vagina during and after labor with saline solutions to which whisky or biochloride of mercury was added," according to a chronicle of the hospital.

The hospital enema was such a standard tool that, for obstetrical purposes, it was often known as the 3H, short for "high, hot, and a hell of a lot." This sort of enema squirted into the rectum soapy water that could cause irritation and other complications.

However, a surprising 1981 British study that randomly assigned midwives and laboring women to an enema or a nonenema group found no difference in the length of labor or in whether the women passed stool during birth. Because the study quickly began to disprove the effectiveness of enemas, the trial concluded early: Midwives, once staunch supporters of enemas, suddenly refused to administer the treatment.

SHAVING

In the nineteenth century, doctors suspected there was dangerous bacteria everywhere: in the air, the sheets, the walls. Even in a woman's pubic hair. After doctors at Harvard and Johns Hopkins published papers in the early 1900s asserting that shaving the area around the vagina could prevent childbed fever—the biggest cause of maternal death at the time—the practice became standard procedure, one most women hated.

In a 1912 letter to the editor of the *Journal of the American Medical Association,* one Oklahoma physician said he would never try to shave a patient's pubic hair, because "In about three seconds after the doctor has made the first rake with his safety [razor], he will find himself on his back out in the yard with the imprint of a woman's bare foot emblazoned on his manly chest, the window sash around his neck and a revolving vision of all the stars in the firmament presented to him. Tell him not to try to shave 'em."

Shaving did not prevent infection. It invited it. The razor often nicked the skin, creating small wounds for germs to enter. The first controlled trial to study whether shaving prevented infection was in 1922, and it found that washing the area with soapy water worked just as well. A 1971 study found that women who were shaved had a 5.6 percent chance of infection, compared with 0.6 percent in those who were not. None of the evidence seemed to matter. Because so many women were having episiotomies, doctors wanted every perineum shaved in case they had to stitch it back together.

Pubic hair shaving, while never popular (new hair growth is uncomfortably itchy), was a controversial topic in the 1970s, a decade that seems to have been all about hair. Feminists and natural-birth advocates considered the act to be dehumanizing, an attack on womanhood, a way of desexualizing the female body, and another outrageous impersonal stamp from an assembly line of hospital rituals. But the practice persisted well into the 1980s. Even as late as 1993, 16 percent of Canadian hospitals still had policies stipulating that women needed to be at least partially shaved when they were admitted for labor. Just in case they needed an episiotomy.

LABOR POSITIONS

Before doctors arrived on the scene, women of the world rarely lay on their backs for birth. Japanese women crawled onto futons, where they were free to find a comfortable position. Jamaican slaves had a birthing tree, often not far from the field where they worked, upon which they would lean during labor. Difficult births called for more unusual positions. A sixteenth-century Italian text recommended dangling a woman's legs over the side of the bed while her rear end was propped over pillows and her head hung backward. Ancient Egyptians sat between bricks. Europeans sat on birth stools. In the early modern period these stools were draped in fabric skirts to hide the woman's buttocks. Sometimes, though, that fabric harbored dangerous bacteria. By the eighteenth century, birth stools had evolved to become taller birth chairs, contraptions that gave doctors more room to manipulate the emerging head.

By the nineteenth century, when doctors were more popular birth attendants, lying down had become so universal among

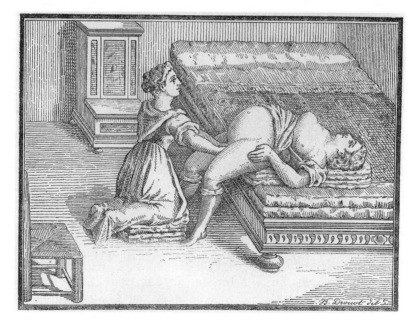

An example of a sixteenth-century Italian labor position. (Courtesy the Wellcome Library)

upper-class women that one European-trained American obstetrician, George Engelmann, was shocked to observe an ancient Peruvian funeral urn decorated with images of a birthing woman sitting on the ground, knees to chest, another woman holding her from behind.

"The method of delivery followed by those, at that time, highly civilized people, a thousand or more years ago, seemed to me so peculiar that I was anxious to know whether other people had similar curious customs and whether any traces of these could be found at the present day," Engelmann wrote on the first page of his classic 1882 text *Labor among Primitive Peoples.* "Moreover, it appeared to me as if a study of obstetric customs among the more primitive people might lead to valuable results which would serve to guide the practice of the present day."

Engelmann conducted a worldwide survey and broke down his findings by geography. In Asia and Africa, squatting and kneeling were very popular, as was sitting on stools and stones. Here's how he described North American practices:

Canada, French settlers. Semi-recumbent on the floor, back against an inclined chair.

Canada, Iroquois. Standing, clinging to the neck [of a helper].

Mexico, Indians, half-breeds, and lower class of whites. Kneeling, clinging to a rope or the neck; squatting; standing, and semi-recumbent on the lap and in bed.

By the end of his research it was clear that Engelmann had become a firm believer in the benefits of delivering in an upright posture. The medical establishment, however, dismissed his work, convinced such positions were beneath proper women. Although kneeling with elbows to the ground could help the birth of a posterior-facing baby, caught from behind, doctors of the enlight-

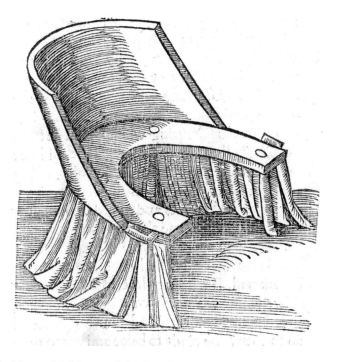

Cloth skirts on birthing stools harbored germs. (Courtesy the Wellcome Library)

enment thought the maneuver was indecent, regardless of how beneficial the pose could be.

In the twentieth century, women gave birth in hospital beds, their arms restrained in wrist cuffs, their legs strapped into stirrups. This position was not just uncomfortable, it was also humiliating. In Russia, as late as the 1980s, delivery beds faced the doors for easy viewing by any passerby. The "maternity houses" were run like factories, with strict rules dictating even when the windows could be opened. Any disobedience would result in punishment.

In hospitals today, laboring women who are not hooked up to epidurals are allowed to wander the halls. They might be encouraged to sit on the toilet—the modern equivalent of a birthing stool—or straddle a large rubber birth ball to help open the cervix.

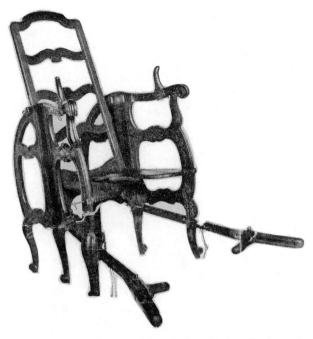

Eighteenth-century French parturition chair, with hand grips. (Courtesy the Wellcome Library)

Yet for the most part, when delivery is imminent, doctors adjust the spotlight, position the splash mat, and order the woman back into bed. The rare exception to this setup is the waterbirth.

WATERBIRTH

Since ancient times, women in warm climates have given birth in oceans and rivers and streams. By 1977, some even were giving birth in an inflatable garden pool under the roof of a state-run hospital in Pithiviers, France. At the time, France was undergoing the same sort of countercultural revolution America was, which made it easier for obstetrician Michel Odent to offer, and women to accept, this new approach.

Odent stumbled on the idea after reading Frederick Leboyer's *Birth without Violence,* a book that advocated immediate gentle baths for newborns as a way of easing their transition into the world. Odent reasoned that if warm baths felt good to infants, they might be of comfort to women during labor. He was right. Women naturally gravitated to the pool, where the water mellowed their labor pain—now called the "aquadural" effect—and helped them relax, which aided dilation. When birth was imminent, most mothers felt an urge to quickly get out of the tub.

"One day, a mother-to-be had not been in water for long when suddenly she had two irresistible contractions and the baby was born before she could feel the need to get out of the pool," Odent recalled. "While giving birth, this woman was really on another planet. It was obvious that in that particular state of consciousness associated with hard labor she miraculously knew that her baby could be born safely under water. There was no panic. It was as if a deep-rooted knowledge could express itself as soon as the intellect was at rest. Occasionally, similar stories happened again. We had learned that a birth underwater is a possibility. A newborn human baby has powerful diving reflexes and is perfectly adapted to immersion."

Igor Charkovsky, a Soviet researcher and swim coach, had come to the same conclusion in 1962, when his daughter, Veta, had been born two months prematurely, weighing only 2.5 pounds. Desperate to help her live, he put her in a tub of warm water, shallow enough for her to lie on the bottom with her head above water, to help strengthen her muscles without stressing them. Eventually, he added more and more water to larger and larger tanks. He gave her live fish and frogs to play with. The baby thrived.

"When she felt hungry she would dive down and pick up a bottle that lay on the bottom of the tank," Charkovsky told one interviewer. "She spent the greater part of her first two years in water. I only took her out of the tank when I was expecting visitors who might be shocked."

Charkovsky was so pleased with the results of his experiment that he came to believe children could be born underwater, nursed underwater, even read to underwater. He launched a training program for pregnant women, instructing them to dunk their heads under water several times a day to reinforce what it feels like to be suspended in amniotic fluid. His unusual physical training went even further, having women do push-ups and splits through their final trimesters.

Eventually, he began orchestrating water deliveries. Yet, despite Charkovsky's years of work on waterbirth, his practices became widely known in the West only after Odent helped to popularize the method.

One of Charkovsky's waterbirth customers was Yekaterina Bagryanskaya, who, in the winter of 1986, reportedly delivered a daughter without pain in a deserted bay of the frigid Crimean Sea, as dolphins splashed around and seagulls screeched overhead. Dolphins, which support each other during labor and help calves to the surface for air—this is why midwives have adopted them as a sort of mascot—have always been a source of mystical inspiration for some people, including Charkovsky, who believed that their aura helped calm mother and baby. Charkovsky also believed in dolphins' ability to detect if something was about to go wrong. Bagryanskaya, however, had no trouble and spent seven hours in the sea with her new daughter over the course of the day. Mother, father, and infant slept that night in a tent on the beach and then walked home three kilometers along craggy cliff paths.

Charkovsky, with no medical training, became an underground cult figure who promoted the belief in waterbirth just as other western countries were embracing alternative birthing methods. Karil Daniels, a filmmaker from San Francisco, went to Moscow in 1984 to film Charkovsky's waterbirths and was impressed by his methods. She included his work in an award-winning documentary she produced called *Water Baby: Experi-*

ences of Waterbirth, and became an enthusiastic champion of waterbirth.

She is less enthusiastic, however, about ocean births.

"I don't feel comfortable with it," she said. "Personally, I feel that one of the great benefits of waterbirth is that mothers can be in control of the birth process. When you're in a wild water environment, many things are out of your control. There may be dangerous things in the ocean or on the beach. I worry about contaminants. You can't control what's in that water and what the temperature is. Years ago I heard about a woman who had an ocean birth with her husband and son nearby, armed with spears in case a shark might come too close. To me ocean birth seems very anxiety producing. But that's the radical edge. There are midwives in Hawaii and Australia and New Zealand who do it."

Although Charkovsky's own popularity diminished in the late 1980s after he showed his British fans a film in which he plunged babies headfirst into a frozen lake, waterbirth had captured mothers' attention.

America's first reported water baby, Jeremy Lighthouse, was born in his parents' San Diego hot tub in 1980. Five years later, Dr. Michael Rosenthal opened the Family Birth Center in the Los Angeles area, offering the country's first institutional setting for waterbirths. In the United Kingdom, companies began renting out portable shallow pools for home births, and women lobbied hospitals to install tubs for the same purpose. Doctors, however, remained wary, citing concerns about waterbirth's safety and questioning exactly how it should be done. What temperature should the water be? Could the mother get overheated? Hypothermic? Would the newborn's body temperature be affected? Would the baby inhale the water? Was there an increased likelihood of infection, especially if the mother's membranes had ruptured? Would it be possible to tell if the mother was bleeding a little or a lot? What about the kinky partner who wanted to jump in the pool naked, as well?

In the midst of this debate, trouble erupted.

In 1992, a Viennese home-birth baby, left underwater for half an hour by its parents, sustained severe brain damage. No professionals had attended the birth. The same year, at a hospital in Bristol, England, a woman who had labored for two and a half hours in warm water delivered a baby that died fifteen hours later. No one sounded an alarm about this hospital death until eighteen months later, when another woman descended into the same tub with tragic consequences. During labor, the midwife noticed the temperature was several degrees above Odent's recommended 99 degrees Fahrenheit. Concerned, she checked the fetal heart rate and found the baby to be in distress. The woman got out of the tub. But the baby's heart rate continued to weaken. Once born, the baby needed resuscitating, and ultimately suffered brain damage. Later, another child born in a tub at a hospital in Oxford died. Then more home waterbirth babies, in Sweden and Moscow, also died.

Although no one could say unequivocally that the water had caused the deaths, the stories were enough to make mothers cool to the idea, at least for a while. Odent said that he never had advocated that women actually give birth under water, and said that in the cases of the deaths, the water temperatures were too hot, the women labored in the pools too long, or infants remained submerged too long after birth.

It is true that babies can be born under water, because they continue to receive oxygen through the umbilical cord. They do not swallow water unless they are born already stressed and oxygen deprived, which causes them to gasp for air. However, as soon as the placenta begins to pull away from the uterine wall, the child's oxygen flow ceases. And because no one can predict exactly when that will happen, the baby should not be held under water after it is born.

Despite the controversy, midwives still believed professionally attended waterbirths had merit. Women said it helped them get through labor without drugs, they felt more in control, and they thought the baby emerged in a more peaceful atmosphere. It also seemed to make pushing easier. In 1995, four natural childbirth advocates, including Beverley Lawrence Beech, organized the First International Water Birth Conference, in Wembley, England. Fifteen hundred midwives, doctors, and parents attended.

"It was really the antagonism from the obstetricians and pediatricians who were saying, 'This is dangerous! You can't do it.' We thought, well, there are thousands of people all over the world having waterbirths. We're going to have to get everybody together to establish what research there is, so that people should know about it and be able to find that research," Beech recalled on the phone from England.

In the early 1990s, about twenty thousand UK women were using the pools. In England alone, eighty hospitals had installed tubs, though many of them were too shallow to be effective. In 1999, the *British Medical Journal* published the first major study of waterbirth. In the four thousand cases examined, five babies died. One fetus was known to be dead before birth; another fatality came from a concealed pregnancy at the end of which the baby was delivered without help in a tub at home. The three other newborn deaths were attributed to a neonatal herpes infection, underdeveloped lungs, and a brain hemorrhage, respectively. Statistically, those deaths translate to 1.2 in a thousand, compared with 0.8 in a thousand low-risk land births. However, only 8 in a thousand water babies needed special care, compared with 9.2 per thousand land-birth babies. Although two of the newborns who died did breathe in water, no deaths were directly attributable to the water.

Regardless of these generally favorable statistics, obstetricians still were not convinced of waterbirth. "Doctors," according to Beech, "still haven't changed their minds." Hospitals offer birthing pools, she explained, but make it difficult for mothers to use them by saying the pool hasn't been cleaned or there's no one there at the moment trained to use it. Most of the British women who try waterbirth—at home or in the hospital—are attended by midwives.

But if the evidence shows waterbirth can be safe and effective, why would doctors throw up obstacles?

"Because it's removing large numbers of women from medical control," replied Beech, honorary chair of the Association for Improvements in the Maternity Services, an English pressure group founded in 1960. "You can't practice a cesarean on a woman having a successful waterbirth. It threatens their practice."

FREEBIRTH

Then there are the women who don't want any medical assistance at all.

Do-it-yourself home birthers often cite historic accounts from Africa or South America or India, where women supposedly give birth alone, squatting in a field before returning to work a couple of hours later. They believe birth should be as simple as it is for animals. In *Unassisted Childbirth*, a 1994 book written by a woman who had four such deliveries at home (sometimes not even her husband was there), author Laura Kaplan Shanley said obstetricians could gain insight from Purina's *Handbook of Cat Care,* which states, "Let her [the cat] walk around [while in labor] and do not insist that she stay in her box."

Loi Medvin believed in giving birth without any interventions, and chose to give birth alone—this was in the mid-1990s—with only the baby's father in attendance. As a twenty-five-year-old living an adventurous gypsy life with her boyfriend, she considered delivering in a hot spring, but ultimately chose otherwise.

"We couldn't find one that I felt I would be comfortable in," she said. "And I didn't want to freak other people out. We ended up at my mom's house in Utah." Her mother is author, midwife, and prenatal yoga expert Jeannine Parvati Baker, whose *Conscious*

Conception: Elemental Journey through the Labyrinth of Sexuality made her a sort of spiritual figure of the feminist movement and an advocate for birth free of the "paid paranoia."

When labor began for Medvin, she and Brian Johnson, the father, were alone in the house. She climbed into the bathtub, and he massaged pressure points on her back and checked her for dilation, although Medvin admits he did not really know what he was doing.

"He did a lot of the reading that I did. He was also in a very trusting place. He most likely could have been a whole lot more educated, but we really were strongly in agreement that this was how we wanted to do it," she recalled.

Her mother, who was supportive, called during labor. Johnson spoke to her on the phone, but Medvin, "in a gray place," tuned out the conversation. When the birth was imminent, she said, she did not really push; her body released the baby. She did tear, which was extremely painful, but she didn't have it stitched, and it healed on its own. Johnson handed the baby to her and, after the placenta came out, they got out of the tub.

Neither knew how to cut or tie the cord, so they left the placenta attached, at the other end of the cord, to their daughter, named Wynn.

"We put the placenta in a lettuce spinner. We had kittens and they were curious and wanted to eat it, so we had to cover it up. I didn't want to introduce any cutting or anything. I wanted to have the birth as whole as possible. I didn't want to cut [the umbilical cord], so I didn't. It fell off four days later."

The practice of not cutting the cord is called a Lotus birth. The baby begins to breathe on its own as soon as the placenta pulls away from the uterine wall.

Medvin said she wasn't scared, but she was in pain "some of the time. . . it was over pretty quick, and really I was too focused to be scared."

Would she do it again?

"I'm definitely an advocate, but I feel like people should really have their baby the way they're more comfortable. Although my mom would say birth is not comfortable. If I did it again, I might just want to have another person there—just to massage me. And I would have us all be more educated."

HYPNOBIRTH

For all those women who don't know how to get to Medvin's "gray place," Marie Mongan offers self-hypnosis.

Mongan's first two birth experiences were of the typically atrocious 1950s-era hospital variety. By the time child number three was due to arrive, in 1959, she told her doctor she would have the baby with no drugs forced on her, no stirrups, no interference, and with her husband by her side—or else she would find another obstetrician. Flabbergasted, the doctor agreed.

By 1987, Mongan, who had a teaching background and was a dean at a women's college, had also become a certified hypnotherapist. During her training, she realized that she had unwittingly used self-hypnosis to birth her third child without pain or fear. If those words sound familiar, it's because Mongan is a modern-day disciple of Grantly Dick-Read. She had read his work and believed in his message. Although Dick-Read said he did not use hypnosis because he thought it would disconnect the woman from her own labor, Mongan believes that when a woman is hypnotized, she still can be fully awake, and in control, perhaps even more alert and aware than at other times.

Shortly after she became a hypnotherapist, Mongan developed a program to help her pregnant daughter use hypnosis so she could give birth without drugs. Since then, she has written a book, trademarked the HypnoBirth name, and launched a worldwide education program that reaches from Singapore to Sweden.

Parents pay between $250 and $350 to take five classes spread over five weeks.

At a recent session in a suburban conference center about an hour west of Boston, reiki masters, doulas, midwives, yoga instructors, nurses, and hypnotherapists from as far away as Tokyo and Dubai had come to hear Mongan, who lives in New Hampshire—the conservative New England state whose motto "Live Free or Die" is punched onto the license plate of every car registered there. She speaks with the authoritative, almost arrogant tone of a radio talk-show host and drops the occasional reference to God. With her short hair and three-button tan suit jacket, she offers all the trappings of a straight-laced grandmother.

But make no mistake: Mongan is a militant when it comes to birth. She refuses to acknowledge that back labor exists—that just puts negative ideas in the mind of laboring women—and corrects the already chastened group when one of them uses the word *delivery*.

"FedEx makes deliveries," she says, "so does UPS." Pregnant women don't.

Birth, she says, is the better word. The only word. In Mongan's world, there are no contractions, just surges and waves. There are no coaches, just "birth companions." The baby is not caught or delivered; it is received or birthed. A due date, she instructs, is a birthing time. Pain, in HypnoBirthing parlance, is nothing more than pressure. Water doesn't break, she says, membranes release. A fetus, she explains, should be called an unborn baby. What Mongan has done is ditch the harsh medical terminology for softer language. The new language is a subtle but powerful way of rejecting the medical model of birth in favor of one that is simple, natural, and not scary.

Her students learn how hypnosis, which helps people stop smoking, stuttering, bingeing, and nail-biting, and eases the discomfort of chemotherapy, can also help women through labor. All they have to do is practice breathing in and tuning out. Follow along: Picture yourself resting on a bed of strawberry-colored mist a foot and a half high. Recite the colors of the rainbow while having your arm softly stroked. Visualize your baby in your arms. Everyone is smiling. This is what a HypnoBirth CD, included in the disseminated packet of relaxation and visualization techniques, instructs pregnant women to do to prepare for birth.

Women in this hypnotic state—what Mongan calls "Lucy/Loosey Limp"—relax using breathing techniques and the power of positive suggestion to influence physiology. Mothers can hear conversation and feel what's going on with their bodies during hard labor, but are able to remain calm and quiet, so much so that attendants can barely tell when, ahem, "surges" are happening. The method also uses light-touch massage to release endorphins—the same feel-good hormones secreted after exercise and sex—as well as physical signals, such as having the birth companion touch the woman's shoulder as a reminder to go more deeply into relaxation.

The effects seem too good to be true. Among all the alternative methods —massage, reflexology, homeopathy, music, white noise, aromatherapy, biofeedback, even magnets—that aim to reduce pain, some studies do offer evidence that hypnosis works best.

DOULAS

Hypnosis is not the only low-tech labor aid proven to be effective. Having another woman present to offer constant reassurance can make birth seem less painful and advance more quickly.

In 1975, American doctors John H. Kennell and Marshall H. Klaus were in Guatemala doing research related to maternal bonding. Because they needed the patients' permission to conduct the study, they sent a female medical student with her clipboard into the room where ten women were expected to labor unattended before being moved to a delivery room. But what happened was startling and completely unexpected.

"She stayed with the moms. Three of them delivered in bed, and three had milk spurting from their breasts" from a surge in oxytocin, the "love" hormone that also causes the uterus to contract, Klaus said. He and Kennell couldn't make sense of the phenomenon. "We said, 'Are the women getting something out of Wendy?'"

Indeed, the student had fouled up their research by remaining with the women after collecting their signatures. Not knowing she shouldn't linger in the labor room, she felt compelled, as a fellow female, to stay, and to soothe and reassure them. Emotional support, the doctors speculated, might actually help labor progress and help the women cope with the pain.

Kennell and Klaus did not even know what to call a woman who was not a midwife but nonetheless gave mothers reassurance during labor. They later heard, in a meeting with the World Health Organization, that in the Middle East, particularly Egypt, women referred to their midwives as "dulas." They also came across the word *doula* in a classic 1970s book on breast-feeding called *The Tender Gift: Breastfeeding*. Doula, in Aristotle's time, meant slave. Greeks used slaves or bondswomen to wet nurse and care for infants. The term later referred to women who helped new mothers with domestic tasks.

Today, a doula is essentially a woman who provides physical and emotional support to a woman in labor by offering words of encouragement, a sip of water, or a massage, staying by the mother's side the whole time, without handling the more technical aspects of the birth.

Klaus and Kennell launched their first real doula study in 1975. The research team had hoped to have twenty normal vaginal deliveries in the doula group and another twenty deliveries in a non-doula group to examine how having support during labor affected mother-child relations right after birth. However, the non-doula group was producing far more complicated deliveries, including a high rate of cesareans. In fact, it took 103 women in the non-doula group to produce just twenty normal vaginal deliveries, compared with only 33 women in the doula group to reach the same target. The linkage seemed clear. And having an uncomplicated birth was not the only benefit the women attended by doulas experienced. They had shorter labors—8.8 hours, compared with the 19.3 hours of the non-doula women. They were also more alert and interactive with their newborns than the women who labored alone.

"Fifteen published studies have shown that if you have a doula, your incidence of a cesarean is reduced 26 percent, and if you have a doula, the birth is 25 percent quicker," Klaus said.

For Klaus, the concept of having continuous emotional support in labor was the missing link in obstetrics. Before midwives fell out of favor, women had the support of other women who knew how and where to touch a laboring woman to ease her pain. They knew what to say. But as women began laboring alone in the hospital, birth seemed to get more complicated, requiring more drugs and more interventions.

In 1992, Klaus and Kennell, along with three nationally respected childbirth experts, formed what's now called DONA International (the DONA having once stood for Doulas of North America) International, turning a concept into a paid profession. In 1994, there were 750 doulas. Today there are over 6,000 worldwide, mostly paid out of pocket by the mothers who hire them.

Still, with so many women now bringing the baby's father with them for the birth, why would anyone need to hire a doula to draw imaginary pictures on her back or whisper encouragement in soothing tones? After studying more than five hundred cases, Kennell found that women who had only their mate in the delivery room had a 22 percent cesarean rate. Those who added a doula to the mix had a 14 percent cesarean rate. This raises the questions: Did nature intend for men to be present at birth? Does a father's own worries add to the anxiety in the room? Does he offer a massage that's more annoying than comforting? Does he interrupt the woman's concentration (such as if he passes out when the epidural needle is stuck into her spine)? Does he inhibit her? Who let the men in to begin with?

8 A FATHER'S PLACE

A GROUP OF pregnant nurses agreed to try giving birth without drugs at the Mayo Foundation in Minnesota. It was the 1940s, and Dr. Robert A. Bradley, who was still training in obstetrics, was studying what happened when husbands were allowed in the labor room for periods of time—though not when the baby actually emerged. He concluded that a spouse's presence seemed to help the laboring mothers relax. When the man left, the woman grew anxious.

Bradley's theory crystallized when one of the women, moments after delivering—as her husband paced in the waiting room—grabbed the doctor to thank him with kisses and hugs.

"Oh, thank you, thank you for showing me how!" she said.

"It hit me like a sledgehammer," Bradley later wrote. "What on earth was this lovely woman kissing me for? Why was I the object of her gratitude as a labor coach while her young lover sat uselessly in the waiting room, fearful and anxious over his sweetheart's safety, eagerly wishing to see the outcome of his love for her, the baby, yet deprived by isolation from the most meaningful emotional experience of their lives together? The more I thought about it, the more ridiculous it seemed."

The Mayo Foundation, like the rest of the medical establishment, thought that having fathers present was a bad idea, mostly out of fear that "outsiders" would contaminate the sterile environment. Who knows how many obstetricians, still almost exclusively men, also feared losing their status to another male in the labor and delivery room. But Bradley persisted. Because he was working at a teaching hospital, he was able to pitch his idea as an experiment, saying a father represented not an additional person in the room, but a substitute for the suddenly unnecessary anesthetist. He also promised to supply the new labor coach with scrubs, cap, and mask similar to those worn by doctors.

In 1962 Bradley published *Father's Presence in Delivery Rooms,* an analysis of his first four thousand cases in which husbands were present throughout the birth as coaches; the doctor's role resembling "that of the lifeguard, who when watching swimmers, did nothing as long as everything was going all right," said Bradley. "With husbands coaching, we have over 90 percent totally unmedicated births. No other approach comes anywhere near that figure."

Bradley, a devout Catholic who grew up on a Kansas farm, was as bombastic as he was folksy, calling the uterus the "baby box" and the clitoris the "passion button." He accepted everything from photographs to food as payment. His critics called him "Barnyard Bradley" because he believed humans could imitate animals in labor and even enjoy unmedicated births. Instead of morphine or scopolamine, Bradley mothers received "PEP," Praise, Encouragement, and assurance of Progress. They also had the baby's father at the foot of the bed, coaching them through their labor. There was a practical side to all of this, of course: Hospital staff—and this is still the case—did not have the time to provide continuous emotional support or instruction to laboring women.

When Bradley died on Christmas day in 1998 at the age of eighty-one, after presiding over nearly twenty thousand unmedicated births, he was known as the "Father of Fathers," a man who had helped western culture overturn thousands of years of tradition that barred fathers from the births of their children.

In some ancient societies, men were considered irrelevant to the birthing cycle; the connection between intercourse and pregnancy was not understood. It was thought that babies were the product of spirits or something the mother ate. Fatherhood, in that sense, was a social construct, not a biological one, and so there was no reason for him to be present during a birth, especially since the mother would be surrounded by practiced women.

But even in places where fathers were recognized as procreators, they were banned from the birth for other reasons. A woman's modesty was sacrosanct. Men were thought to be unclean and dangerous. Having a male witness birth was considered immoral, repugnant, and, frankly, stupid. What, women wondered, could men know that a female midwife didn't? And why would males want to be there? In 1522, believing it important that he witness a birth, a Dr. Wertt of Hamburg snuck from confinement to confinement dressed as a woman until a midwife realized he was a man and raised the alarm. His deception did not go over well, and he was burned to death, with other physicians watching, no doubt reinforcing for them that birth had been, and should always be, the exclusive realm of females.

Except for the rare man who hoped to edify himself, males routinely stayed away. Yet fathers were not always disengaged: They had their own rituals and chores, building birth huts, tending fires, and protecting the physical or spiritual space during labor. The Ainu men of Japan meditated on fatherhood for twelve days in seclusion, during which they gave their soul to the child as the mother gave her body. The Arapesh men of New Guinea bathed in aromatic oils to purify and anoint the entry into fatherhood. And on the Trobriand Islands in the South Pacific, the father stood guard with a spear outside the hut to protect his woman from "prowling sorcerers," who were actual men skulking around as part of a birth rite.

In many places, it wasn't just that the father was excluded from a birth; often he was physically isolated from the mother and child. On Lukunor, another island in the South Pacific, men left their wives when labor started and slept and ate with other men for a month, at all times keeping a distance from the birth hut. The same was true on the Micronesian island of Kosrae, where the man was banished for months after the baby arrived, so that neither mother nor child caught a disease from him. On New Guinea, men were not allowed to see their wives from the moment labor began until one month later, when a big public feast introduced the baby to all, including its father. After the feast, mother and child retreated to the birthing hut—sans father—for a year of seclusion. Even in eighteenth-century England, women were not allowed to see their husbands for the entire month-long stay at a lying-in hospital.

There were, however, a few places where men were central to births. On Yap, a spit of an island in the South Pacific between Guam and New Guinea, the father was the normal birth attendant. So, too, on Easter Island, far off the coast of Chile. Among the Huichol tribe of Mexico, in order to make the father a partner in the mother's pain, a string would be tied around his testicles; the mother would pull the tether as each contraction peaked. In Ireland, Scotland, and parts of India, men wore women's clothes to symbolically assume some of the pain. In other places, women kept the father's pants or hat nearby as a good luck charm.

In Europe, however, men rarely were allowed into the birth chamber. If they were, it was only because the midwife needed his strength to hold the mother while she pushed or to help force out the baby. In extreme circumstances, midwives instructed men to mount their wives in an effort to lubricate and open the birth canal. Even Aristotle said that although parents should avoid sex during pregnancy, they should have intercourse just before the birth to "shake up the child and bring it out more easily." Guillemeau, a seventeenth-century French physician, revived the practice of sex during labor. There is most likely a connection between that directive and the era's common belief that the white sticky coating of vernix that covers newborns was actually the father's sperm. Yet sex often worked, because, as modern science now knows, sperm contains prostaglandin, a hormone that helps the cervix open.

MODERN MAN

As hospital births became common in the last century, men were removed even further from the process. They would drop off their wives at the admissions desk and go back to work or back home to bed. They hunted, took in ball games, and mowed the lawn while the women cursed, cried, and contracted. Sometimes, with no place to go, they hung around hospital hallways for news. Eventu-

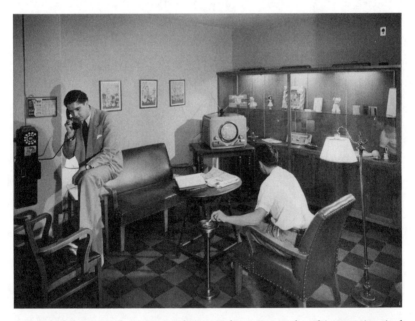

A *"stork club" at Wesley Memorial Hospital. (Courtesy the Chicago Historical Society)*

ally, as hospital facilities expanded and modernized, expectant fathers could be found sitting on the edge of a seat in the "stork club"—specially designed waiting areas near the maternity ward where fathers could take off their suit jackets, fret, smoke, talk on a pay phone, listen to the radio, and, later, watch TV. As late as the 1970s, some stork clubs kept "father books," blank journals in which men, trying to fill the anxious hours, could write the news of their babies, reveal their fears about labor and delivery, and thank the "golden hands" of the doctor.

"Stork club empty," one lonely man wrote in 1952 while waiting for his wife to deliver at Wesley Memorial Hospital in Chicago. "God and I are keeping a vigil." Another new father that same year wrote: "This is the fourth girl born . . . anybody got a suggestion on how to get a boy?"

At the time, Chicago Board of Health regulations allowed men to see their wives only briefly during labor and never during delivery. Such was standard practice in hospitals just about everywhere. But attitudes about paternal involvement slowly were changing.

In 1946, Virginia Mason Hospital in Seattle allowed fathers to stay for the birth as long as the mother had caudal anesthesia, which would keep her in bed, calm and pain free—an easier birth for a father to witness. In 1953, Mount Sinai Hospital in New York City began inviting fathers to participate in prenatal classes, which included a demonstration on how to give newborns a bath and explained how to prepare baby formula, "an important part of baby care which some of the wives suggested as handy for their husbands to learn."

Still, by 1961, only half of all fathers at Mount Sinai were remaining with their wives during labor—and none during delivery. Why? Such was hospital policy, but witnessing birth was also a new experience for a rather conservative generation of men, and many found it difficult. "Sometimes it looks like their hair is actually standing up straight," Mary Jane Sherritt, the hospital's supervisor of maternity, said of the husbands' reactions.

Of course, there were some men who, regardless of hospital restrictions, would not leave before delivery. They wanted to see their babies born, and they wanted to support and protect their wives. This was especially true when the woman was having a child after a previous harsh birth, when they might have been strapped down or forced to take drugs they did not want. How could any of that happen if the father was in the room?

"Girls who cried were told to blame their husbands for the agony they were in," Robert W. Goldfarb told the *Ladies' Home Journal* in 1958, recalling his wife's first delivery three years earlier, during which she had been strapped down and left alone in the hospital. "Muriel told me that during the final stages of labor some of these girls did scream bitterly against their husbands. Yet these men were waiting in their own anguish for some news of their wives. Muriel didn't blame me for her pain, yet I knew what she had endured would scar her deeply, perhaps forever."

When it was time for the second Goldfarb child to be born, Muriel insisted that Robert be there. The obstetrician said he believed the board of health would prohibit it. But when Muriel called the board of health, she found there wasn't any such regulation. The doctor reluctantly consented.

"Muriel and everyone else who knew I would be with her kept asking about my feelings toward her once the birth was over," Robert recalled. "Would I find her less attractive after seeing her raised so awkwardly? She'd be swabbed and decked with sterile sheets. Would I ever think of her as romantic and pretty again? I wondered, too, though I don't believe I ever admitted it. I know this now. Those few minutes in the delivery room made her more beautiful and made me love her more than ever before."

Yet the Goldfarbs' ability to stay together during birth in the late 1950s was exceptional—on both sides of the Atlantic.

In 1961, the year before men were allowed into English delivery rooms, the *British Medical Journal* published a letter from a man saying fathers should have a right to remain for births and that the "pathetic chain-smoking, restless, and flower offering expectant father should be a figure of the past." Not everyone agreed. A -doctor from Northern Ireland said that if hospitals caved to such requests, they would be pandering "to morbid curiosity and sensationalism" that would further encourage "a highly unnatural trend with the mumbo-jumbo of pseudopsychology. The proper place for the father, if not at work, is the 'local' [the corner pub], whither instinct will usually guide him."

Another doctor responded with unusual frankness by saying,

> The periodic distention of the vulva, the accompanying discharge of faeces and urine, and the public exposure of parts usually described as private do not make an edifying spectacle, and one sometimes wonders how a husband who has watched all this can ever have intercourse with his wife again. And, apart from the aesthetic shock, the witnessing of an episiotomy, a perineal laceration, a brisk hemorrhage or the resuscitation of an asphyxiated baby may have dire physical results in a layman sitting masked and gowned in the atmosphere of the delivery rooms. . . . [It is] a sadistic and unnatural curiosity.

Why would anyone want to see such a "disgusting miracle"?

In America, hospital resistance was fierce well into the mid-1960s. The progressive Yale–New Haven Hospital rejected the plea from one of its own doctors to witness his wife's delivery of triplets in 1965. The decision was especially difficult for the father, as he had attended the birth of his first child in California, where doing so was legalized in 1964.

As natural childbirth became more popular, and more fathers were needed to time contractions and help the woman focus through her pain, men began to challenge—and sometimes disregard—hospital policy. In 1964, New Jersey father John O. Keim was fined $150 for gaining unauthorized entry to the delivery room to see the birth of his second child. He was charged with disorderly conduct for refusing to leave his wife's side. John Quinn, a California college student, chained himself to his wife while she was in labor to protest the hospital's ban on his being in the room. The police were called. He made headlines.

In the early 1970s, Evelyn and Bruce Fitzgerald, a married couple from Valparaiso, Indiana, took their indignation one step further. They had practiced Lamaze during pregnancy and wanted to be together throughout the birth. When their local public hospital refused, the Fitzgeralds sued, claiming their constitutional rights, including their right to privacy as a married couple, were being violated. The district court disagreed with them. The couple lost their appeal after the hospital administrator argued that there was no place for husbands to change from street clothes into sterile scrubs, and therefore the men could increase the danger of infection and disrupt delivery room routine. The ruling stated that "individual hospitals should be permitted to make individual choices, rather than having an inflexible rule imposed upon all hospitals in the nation by federal judicial decision."

By the time of that decision, however, most hospitals had changed their policies and were permitting parents to stay together—with two exceptions: those who weren't married and those whose babies were born by cesarean. In the mid-1970s, only a few hospitals allowed fathers in the operating room, and even then, the couples were granted permission case by case. Some hospitals approved only those who had taken special classes that involved slides of an actual cesarean and warnings about what to expect.

It took unmarried couples even longer to change policies. In 1982, Mercy-Memorial Hospital in Michigan told Edward Coch he could not be with Karen Whitman when she had their baby because they were not husband and wife and hospital policy allowed only a woman's immediate family to be with her during delivery. Stunned, they took the hospital to court, lost initially, and then won on appeal. All in time for the birth.

"Now we can have the baby together, the way we want it," Whitman said after the decision.

Today, of course, the man standing next to the bed does not need to be the woman's husband or lover. He can be the sperm donor. He can be one of two daddies about to adopt the child. Or perhaps he's just a friend. Indeed, once political gravity began drawing men into the birth room, it did not matter who they were.

PUT ME IN, COACH

At the end of the 1960s, only 15 percent of men were attending the births of their children. By the late 1970s, a majority of men were participating right up until the cord cutting. They had to. It was now their duty. No longer mere husbands and fathers, the natural childbirth movement transformed IBM executives and ironworkers into labor and delivery coaches. To qualify for the position, they put humility aside, sat atop pillows on Lamaze class floors, and practiced counting and breathing exercises.

Bradley fathers cheered their women to "Push! Push!" the way Vince Lombardi told his centers to hold the line. In Lamaze classes, instructors would counsel fathers-to-be with boxing metaphors. "She will want to quit. She will want to throw in the towel. You must urge her on."

Men did urge on their women, some more successfully than others. Though vast numbers tried to focus their partner's breathing, not all succeeded. Throughout the 1970s and even into the 1990s, men said they were happy to experience something as profound as birth. But they increasingly found they weren't just coaches. They also were protectors and referees, helping to ensure that the birth played out the way the woman wanted it to.

"It doesn't matter how much pain I'm in, don't let me succumb to drugs!" wives told their husbands before labor started. Such instructions put men in an even more uncomfortable spot. Guys wanted to be supportive, but had no real tools to help.

"I had seen my wife cry before, I had seen her in pain, but never like that, gripping the bed railing, her muscles straining, her face convulsed," a *New York Times* reporter, whose own father was at a classical music concert when he had been born in 1948, wrote in 1984 under the headline "Doubts in the Delivery Room":

> It is never easy to watch someone you love suffer, but it seemed particularly cruel to join her doctor in denying her requests for a sedative until the final minutes. That was my job. In natural childbirth, the role of the father during labor is to help his wife manage the pain as contractions intensify. Try telling your wife that, ultimately, despite efforts to keep her mind off labor, the only thing you can do to relieve the worst pain she's ever experienced is to coach her on breathing fast and wipe her brow periodically with a wet washcloth. . . . I think the problem is that natural childbirth forces a man to live suspended somewhere among the roles of husband, lover, partner, protector and father, not knowing which way to turn.

Some men found themselves arguing with the staff, or found that their touch or words of encouragement annoyed their wives as labor intensified.

"Since the birth I've found that many of my male friends have had similar experiences," anthropologist Richard Reed wrote in *Mothering* magazine in 1996. "We see ourselves as companions in a sacred experience, but our partners often think we are distant, combative, or unaware of their needs. . . . I asserted myself in the most stereotypical male manner. I complained to the nurse about the questions, argued when they strapped on the fetal monitor, and even blocked the doorway when a nurse came to take away the natural birthing bed. Finally, my belabored wife asked me to stop my fighting."

All of this hand-wringing led to the question: "Was it time to fire the coach?"

A 1992 study asked fathers in the San Francisco area who were present for birth: Were they coaches, teammates, or witnesses? Most men said they ended up being witnesses. Being anything more, at a time of so much turmoil, was too much to ask.

"Labor coaches—the term rankles," one father wrote:

At its root is a desire to provide men with an easy and appealing access to the sacred circle. They like sports. Call them coaches, and they will feel at home in the labor room. Coaches are take-charge guys, in control, men who make important decisions and always keep an eye on the scoreboard. Above all, coaches focus on the outcome— achievement, victory, success. The term is not only misleading; it also grants false entry into the circle and, worse, fosters the very attitudes that alienate men from participating more fully in the ritual of birth.

In truth, it was epidurals that made the coaching irrelevant. With the woman resting comfortably while her uterus did all the work, fathers could also relax, or fetch ice chips.

Maybe that's enough to expect. Anthropologist Wenda Trevathan believes there's good reason to keep fathers engaged in the room, even if it's just to experience—and not participate in—

the birth. "In today's highly mobile nuclear families, child care by the father may be the only relief the mother has; thus it is adaptive to enhance his interest and confidence in infant caretaking by allowing him to attend the birth of the child."

THE COUVADE SYNDROME

In other cultures, fathers *have* had a specific role—one very similar to the mothers': They act as if they're in labor and after the baby is born, they "lie-in," sometimes with the postpartum mother taking care of them. Two thousand years ago, in Corsica, the woman did not rest postpartum; she waited on the father as if he were the one who had suffered. Marco Polo observed that in China, the husband was put to bed for forty days with the newborn beside him. Among the Arapesh of New Guinea, it was the father who received congratulations and presents after a birth.

These practices are considered *couvade,* from the French *couver,* to hatch. Some *couvade* customs forbade men from smoking, bathing, eating certain foods, tying knots, or venturing outside for long stretches. Dinka fathers in Sudan had to remain in the birth hut for several days to help "nurse" the new babies. And in South America, men cut themselves with animal teeth to feel pain, painted themselves with red dye to mimic blood, and hung in their hammocks for days moaning, sweating, and straining as if they were giving birth.

Since the early days of anthropology, there have been many theories about the origins and meaning of *couvade.* Some said the practice was a male expression of jealousy, a cry for attention, or a reflection of their ambivalence about the birth. Others believed that these actions were a way for the man to show he identified with the mother, proof of a mystical link between the parents. A few speculated that it was women who invented *couvade* to keep their men close to home where they were needed, or to engender sympathy by making the father feel pain through a restricted diet or restricted freedoms.

Today, psychologists believe real physiological *couvade* symptoms reflect how highly connected men are to their pregnant partners. In the early 1980s, doctors began noticing that expectant fathers in western cultures were increasingly developing the same bloat, weight gain (ten pounds on average), fatigue, insomnia, indigestion, insatiability, irritability, restlessness, and urge to scrub the house as the expectant mothers. However, with a popular culture that was demanding paternal participation from the moment the Early Pregnancy Test revealed those two parallel lines confirming conception, it's possible that it wasn't a matter of more men experiencing *couvade* symptoms—they were just more willing to admit that they, too, indulged in pickles and ice cream for nine months.

No one is sure exactly how many fathers exhibit *couvade* symptoms. In 1982 researchers reported that of the more than 200 -fathers-to-be they studied in the New York area, 22 percent needed treatment for nausea, vomiting, cramps, and toothaches, symptoms that were not there prior to the pregnancy and disappeared with the birth. Almost all of the sufferers were first-time fathers. A 1985 study of 147 expectant fathers in the Milwaukee area found 90 percent of the men had multiple *couvade* symptoms, including insomnia, fatigue, weight changes, and irritability.

Other studies have indicated that the phenomenon is not merely psychosomatic. Blood and saliva samples from expectant dads do show hormonal shifts that reflect changes similar to those the mother is experiencing. Testosterone levels drop, and estrogen levels rise. The stress hormone cortisol and the milk inducing hormone prolactin also increase in the weeks before birth as the men prepare to become fathers. Some men say they even feel sick to the point of vomiting after birth, whether it's an adrenaline letdown or some sign of empathy.

But there are other plausible explanations for many of these symptoms. For example, pregnant women don't have room for large meals in their squished stomachs, so they need to eat small portions, more frequently. Men are likely to eat along with them but being able to eat larger portions, they gain weight. In the last trimester, many women are too uncomfortable to sleep, and if they're thrashing around in bed, the men are probably waking up, as well. As for those hormonal changes, researchers say it's synchronization between two intimate people, just like the well-known phenomenon of women who are together every day (sisters, nuns, even coworkers) tending to menstruate at the same time every month.

Whether men experience *couvade* or not, there are plenty of other birth rituals for them to partake in: sitting through prenatal classes, going to ultrasound appointments, strapping on thirty-pound lead empathy bellies, attending coed baby showers, making small talk during epidural insertions, photographing the birth, cutting the umbilical cord, changing diapers, handling the 2:00 a.m. feeding, taking paternity leave, or building an addition on the house. Should that be the extent of their involvement?

In 1960, a doctor toiling at Middlesex Hospital in West London interviewed fathers and their partners a couple of months after delivery. He asked the men if they were happy to have been present during the birth. They said yes, almost without exception.

That doctor, George Davidson, then spoke to the fathers alone and assured them that the questions and answers were confidential and that he had no strong views himself. This time, most of the men said that although the birth was a remarkable experience, it was one they could have missed. Many felt it did not improve their relationship with their wives, and some said they had a hard time putting the birth image out of their mind when it was time for sex. Looking back on that study, it sounds as if men, though willingly going into the delivery room, were still uncomfortable there.

That study was long forgotten, pushed aside by the family-centered childbirth movement that, in addition to bringing dads bedside, brought siblings into the delivery room. Then in the late 1990s, waterbirth pioneer Michel Odent did something that seemed even more radical than advocating babies be born in water. He stayed out of the delivery room when his partner gave birth to their son. Despite all the babies he had caught, he did not want to distract his mate from her primal act or spoil their sexual relationship.

Odent, who now lives in England and runs his Primal Health Research Centre in London, had interviewed couples years after their babies had been born to research how the birthing event shaped their lives together. He found that having the father there is not always best. In the short term, Odent believes, men can actually hinder labor and may be contributing to the soaring cesarean rate. When a father is distressed seeing the woman in pain, he might try to talk rationally to her, in a conversation that could go something like this:

Are you all right? What's going on?

I'm having a CONTRACTION! Stop! Talking!

Such chatter, Odent says, forces the woman to respond with the rational part of her brain, and that's very distracting for someone who needs to be in touch with her primitive self. In 2000, when he was publicizing his latest book, *The Scientification of Love,* he offered little proof but said the anecdotal material was remarkable. "The labour may be going slowly, slowly, and suddenly, for some unexpected reason, the man has to go out" of the room, he told one newspaper. "As soon as he is gone, the woman starts to scream and shout, and when he comes back, the baby has been born. I have many stories where the woman says everything was wonderful but unfortunately my husband was not there. It is as if women have two languages. They are convinced they cannot give birth without the participation of the baby's father. But on the day of the birth, they said something different with their body language."

Odent also believes that having the father witness the birth can strain the couple's sex life. "I have seen so many couples who had wonderful births according to the present criteria, yet several years later they divorced," he said. "They have remained good friends, but they are not sexual partners anymore."

Odent's views, while intriguing, are also extreme given that most maternity systems in industrialized countries today are geared toward having fathers present—even employing them to cut the cord. It's now difficult for fathers to opt out, regardless of how squeamish they are. In one recent case, a father said he could not bear to watch his fiancée have a cesarean. For different reasons than a man might have had two hundred years ago, he tried to stay away from the birth scene, but he could not entirely escape. Hospital staff led him out of the operating room into another chamber nearby, where the surgery was broadcast on a closed-circuit television.

9   THE POSTPARTUM PERIOD

THE BABY IS born. But the work is not done. The mother's uterus continues to contract to expel the placenta and shrink to its original size. Meanwhile, someone has to cut the cord and dress the stump. The placenta has to be inspected and disposed of. The mother needs to rest, and, of course, the newborn must be fed. But different cultures have had very different methods for addressing each of these actions. Throughout history, the immediate postpartum period has been as much a victim of fashion and misconception as has labor and birth. And standard practice still varies among countries, hospitals, doctors, and midwives.

The first act that usually occurs after the slippery baby emerges is the cutting of the umbilical cord. The cord, obviously, must be severed to free the baby from its mother. The act also forces the newborn to breathe air through its lungs for the first time. Perhaps because of the symbolism of that moment, cord cutting has been a magnet for drama, ceremony, and superstition.

Since antiquity, midwives have cut the cord with whatever tools were available: sharpened stones, seashells, bamboo, glass, even thin hard crusts of bread. Some slashed the cord without first tying a string around it, believing the blood should drain from the baby so as not to poison it, though doing so could prove fatal. In eighteenth-century France, midwives thought such "draining" could even prevent smallpox. Louise Bourgeois, the famous French midwife, tied the cord to the mother's leg before the placenta was expelled out of fear that the afterbirth would retreat further into the womb and choke her.

In other cultures, midwives have left the cord stump longer for boys, to give the penis something to mimic. Some thought longer stumps gave children good singing voices. In remote villages in India, midwives waited as much as twenty minutes before severing the cord. Depending upon the trade common among their caste, they might use a sharp trowel, a saw-tooth sickle, a leather worker's knife, or scissors, and dress the cord stump with a mixture of cow dung, straw, and dirt. There was a 14 percent death rate among newborns in these Indian villages, according to a study published in 1965. Tetanus was the greatest killer, the infection having direct access to the child through its navel.

In most hospitals today, cutting the cord is such an uneventful routine that it can pass unnoticed by the overwhelmed mother. Doctors generally wait about thirty seconds, a time period long enough, they believe, for the baby to receive all the blood it needs from the placenta. (There is some concern that allowing too much blood to flow from the placenta can raise the infant's blood pressure.) They then apply two clamps, break out the scissors, and often ask the father if he wants to cut between the ligatures. Doing all of this quickly also allows for the baby to be suctioned, weighed, and swaddled, before it gets cold.

Some childbirth experts argue that, rather than being guided by a clock, it's best to wait until the cord stops pulsing before cutting, allowing the baby to receive all the blood it was meant to receive from the placenta. They say that helps the mother, as well, because the placenta shrinks as it pumps out the extra blood, making it easier to deliver.

Not surprisingly, midwives and doctors have been arguing for centuries about the timing. It's nearly impossible to say who's right. An impartial source is England's Cochrane Database, which tracks and reviews evidence-based medical information, including that related to childbirth. The database looks at all of the studies, sorts the good ones from the bad, and puts the findings together in a neat summary. In the case of cord cutting, the database declares, "Optimal timing for clamping of the umbilical cord at birth is unclear. Early clamping allows for immediate resuscitation of the newborn." But, the report continues, "Delaying clamping may facilitate transfusion of blood between the placenta and the baby." That blood flow helps get the lungs going, especially in preterm babies, who have the most difficulty with respiration. Delaying cord cutting even 30 to 120 seconds helps babies born before thirty-seven weeks adjust to their new surroundings.

At the other end of the umbilicus is the placenta, which, at term, is purplish red and weighs about one-sixth of the baby. (Identical twins share one large placenta, though each has its own cord.)

No doubt impatient after hours, even days, of labor, midwives and doctors have tried all sorts of ways to detach the afterbirth from the uterus and have it expelled more quickly. Hippocrates advised giving sneezing powder to the mother while holding her mouth and nostrils closed. Ancient Greeks placed the newborn—still attached to the cord—on a leather pillow filled with air, which was pricked and slowly deflated, gently tugging on the cord above. The most antsy attendants gave the cord a good yank, often on the false belief that the womb was about to clamp shut, preventing expulsion. That practice, which could lead to fatal hemorrhage, could pull the uterus out as well. North American Indians used "squaw belts," which were wrapped around the mother's midsection and pulled tight. The Chinese (who believed the placenta was a fetal pillow) stepped on the mother's belly.

Once the placenta was expelled, birth attendants usually inspected it to make sure there were no little bits still inside the uterus to cause infection. If the placenta was whole, doctors and midwives were then faced with the decision of how to dispose of it.

Most mammals, from monkeys to pigs to cats to mice, eat the placenta. This is known as placentaphagy. Even some herbivores, such as goats, consume the organ. These animals—it's almost always the mother—eat it compulsively, even before attending to the offspring. Scientists believe one evolutionary reason for gorging on the organ is that the mother does not want the scent of the afterbirth to attract predators. Another reason could be that new mothers are hungry and the placenta is full of nutrients that can give a quick boost to a female about to start nursing. Furthermore, the organ is coursing with oxytocin, which if ingested, can help prevent postpartum hemorrhage.

Among more than three hundred human cultural groups in the world, very few are known to eat the afterbirth. On Java and Kol, women ate it to boost fertility. In Transylvania, a woman who did not want more children burned the placenta and put the ashes in her husband's drink. In the Philippines, midwives would add placenta blood to porridge to improve the new mother's strength. And throughout Asia, from Vietnam to Burma, the placenta was dried and used for medicinal purposes.

Few in America eat the afterbirth, although it has been done. In the 1970s, placentaphagy became part of radical home birth customs, particularly in the San Francisco area. One 1980 estimate in *Science Digest* said 5 percent of such West Coast deliveries involved consuming the afterbirth; the East Coast rate among home-birthers was about 1 or 2 percent. It is unclear how many of the placentaphagists were vegetarians, but probably many were. They considered the placenta to be sacred, and, of course, because the organ gave life and nothing was killed to put it on the table, it was considered an honor to consume it.

"The mother ate some raw first; and then let me take some into the kitchen for fixing," Jeannine Parvati wrote in her 1978 book *Hygieia: A Woman's Herbal*. "This meat still felt very much alive to me as I began to slice it and sauté it in garlic and oil. . . .

By the time the placenta was tender, the birthday party members were very hungry, and exhausted. After the supper, eaten in a glowing silence, everyone was energized, very much re-vitalized. . . . Notwithstanding, the first time I ate placenta has also been my last time. . . . Guess I just lost [the] taste." Parvati instructed readers to pause before eating placenta to "let it speak," and chew it slowly: "Placenta is a rare privilege for most of us."

Still not everyone knew exactly the best way to eat it. In 1983, *Mothering* magazine offered help, publishing placenta recipes such as these:

PLACENTA COCKTAIL
¼ raw placenta

8 ounces of V-8 juice

2 ice cubes

½ carrot

blend for 10 seconds at high speed

PLACENTA PIZZA TOPPING
Grind placenta.

Sauté in 2 tbs. olive oil w/ 4 garlic cloves

Add: ¼ tsp. fennel, ¼ tsp. pepper, ¼ tsp. paprika, ¼ tsp. salt,

½ tsp. minced onion, ½ tsp. oregano, ¼ tsp. thyme and ¼ cup wine.

Allow to stand 30 min., then add to pizza.

Contemporary placenta eating continues. In 1998, British celebrity chef and new dad Hugh Fearnley-Whittingstall fried a woman's fresh afterbirth in oil with garlic, turned it into pâté, and served it to dinner guests for a television cooking segment. In 1999, a Hong Kong newspaper reported that a syndicate arranged for people to visit the mainland to eat human placenta sashimi, believed to be good for health and beauty. Although many Chinese herbalists prescribe dried powdered placenta, called *ziheche,* usually made from the afterbirths of pigs, doctors have condemned the idea of eating uncooked human organs because doing so could spread disease, such as AIDS or hepatitis.

But who could resist trying it? Even its name connotes gourmand potential: *Placenta* is a Latin word for cake. Gabriele Fallopio, or Fallopius, who published anatomical observations in mid-sixteenth-century Venice, named the organ. He also named the vagina. You might think he named the fallopian tubes, but he actually called them *uteri tuba;* others would eventually name the tubes after him. In France, the placenta was called the loaf, tart, or biscuit. Placenta: the *other* bun in the oven.

Whether people eat the organ or not, they almost always handle the placenta with care, assign it spiritual qualities, or believe it affects the life of the child. In the golden era of anthropology, researchers noted that the !Kungs called the placenta the "older sister"; Muslims referred to it as "the twin"; Japanese children were supposed to laugh while it was buried so the infant would be happy; Thais washed it in a pot with salt in hopes that the baby would not get pimples; Iranians stuffed it in mouse holes hoping to make the child smart; and Mexicans placed it in a tree, thinking it would make the child a good climber. In the Marshall Islands, a boy's placenta would have been thrown into the sea to make him an expert fisherman.

Few cultures have thrown out the placenta. Although many western hospitals today incinerate the organ as medical waste, some maternity facilities send them to researchers or cosmetic makers. Between 1975 and 1992, for example, placentas from 282 British hospitals, weighing 360 tons, were collected by Merieux UK Ltd., a subsidiary of a French pharmaceutical company.

"We use placentas from normal, healthy births only. Placenta is an extremely valuable and rare resource which, instead of being wasted, is used to make pharmaceutical products," Michael O'Gorman, a Merieux manager, told the London *Times* in 1992 when Harrods was selling a £20 vial of RoC face cream— a major brand—with human placenta that supposedly moisturized and regenerated the skin. "Selling placenta is illegal," O'Gorman explained. "Our arrangement is that we pay a donation to the hospital of £5 a box and each box holds 15 to 20 pounds. The money usually goes to labour wards. I believe one bought an underwater birthing bath."

In Japan, where placentas traditionally have been stored in ritual vessels, manufacturers in the early 1990s began adding placenta to beverages, such as those called "Vita X." If that was not enough of a rejuvenator, people could buy a thirty-milliliter (one-ounce) skin lotion product, also made from human placenta extract, which was rich in vitamins, minerals, amino acids, and other health-enhancing substances. The lotion cost ten thousand yen, about ninety dollars.

In 2001, dozens of cosmetic companies informed the U.S. Food and Drug Administration of their use of human placenta. Even Frédéric Fekkai on Rodeo Drive has offered Oscar week European Plasma facials. A key ingredient: afterbirth.

LYING-IN

Of course, there is another postpartum beauty secret that is too often overlooked: sleep.

The first days and weeks at home with a new baby should ideally be calm, restful, and private, and traditional lying-in customs encouraged just that. Almost every culture had elaborate rites to encourage women to remain confined, with their babies, for a set period of time. Mayan mothers, for example, did not resume their normal duties for twenty days, and Japanese women remained in the birth chamber for three weeks after delivery.

221

Until birth moved to the hospital, keeping mothers and babies huddled quietly helped establish breast-feeding success and forge a bond. But there were other reasons to keep them together in isolation. Some cultures believed that women were in grave danger in the weeks just after delivery, susceptible to everything from blood clots to evil spirits; they confined the mother and child so as to protect them. In southeastern Nepal, people believed ghosts could invade the open "sore" of the birth passage and cause madness or infertility; so women there stayed in a shuttered room for six days. In India, the length of a Hindu woman's lying-in depended on her caste.

In Europe and many other places, postpartum women were once considered polluted and therefore dangerous to men; so new mothers were not allowed to prepare or cook food for forty days. Luckily, God-sibs were there to help. In England, women stayed confined for as long as a month, a celebratory time with mothers being fed special caudles and cocooned among her friends, outside the company of men. (Fathers called this time their "gander month.") The women marked the changing of bed linens in a ceremony called "the upsitting," after which the mother would rest for another ten days before moving freely inside the house. Even England's early maternity hospitals required 30-day confinements.

Whether at home or in the hospital, the British postpartum period would officially end with a "churching," a new mother's first trip outside. For that rite—a custom that persisted until the 1950s—she donned a veil, and, surrounded by her midwife and God-sibs as a means of "social enclosure," she went to church and settled into the "uprising seat," a special pew that accommodated all of the women. Initially, churching was a purification rite, similar to the Jewish restriction against women entering temple for thirty-three days after the birth of a son or sixty-six days after the birth of a daughter. But after the sixteenth century, the Protestant ceremony became a simple ten-minute thanksgiving for surviving the ordeal of birth. The minister would recite a psalm and the Lord's Prayer and then accept an offering of a few pence for himself and the parish clerk.

Throughout the Victorian era, obstetric textbooks warned that mothers could be struck with blood clots or uterine prolapse if they walked too soon after birth, and recommended nine straight days of bed rest, especially for the upper class who were thought to be more susceptible to illness.

"Just because some leather-nerved and slow-witted woman can go through a childbirth and be back at work the next day, or even on the afternoon of the same day. . . the impression has become prevalent that a woman is justified in getting up and resuming her duties just as soon as she feels able or inclined," a doctor wrote in *Good Housekeeping* in 1914. "By the mercy of heaven, a considerable majority of women, particularly those of the more intelligent and highly developed types, are so prostrated by the physical strain and suffering that they are perfectly willing, of their own accord, to lie at rest for a reasonable length of time. . . . It is literally as unsafe, and as utterly impermissible, for a woman to stand—let alone move about and work and lift weights—short of ten or fifteen days after her *accouchement*, as it would be for her to attempt to walk on a broken leg within the same period."

By 1937, two weeks had become the standard lying-in period for hospital births in Europe and North America; mothers were kept in bed and fed food fit for an invalid. But the outbreak of World War II created hospital crowding, and staff suddenly were scrambling to free up beds. They sent mothers home sooner, sometimes within a day, and new studies were showing it was safe for them to do so. A 1944 study in the *Journal of the American Medical Association* reported that women allowed to walk around within three or four days of birth had no uterine prolapse or blood clots and were generally healthier than those who stayed in bed ten to twelve days, which actually made them *more* prone to clotting.

When childbirth centers first hit the scene in the 1970s, many women said the best part of delivering there was how quickly they could leave for home. A baby born before noon could be nestled in its own bedroom before 10:00 p.m. the same day. In an era when women did not want to be stuck in the hospital, such results were hailed as progress.

"Postnatal hospital stays are decreasing in length not only because insurance companies have begun to assess why childbirth is so expensive, but also because of a movement of women across this country who don't want childbirth treated as an illness and have welcomed the opportunity to leave the hospital as soon as possible. Yet hospitals have for decades encouraged women to stay," wrote Alexandra Lally Peters, a former president of the Maternity Center Association, in a letter to the editor of the *New York Times* in 1994. "Because these women, who aren't really sick and who require minimal care, are paying plenty for their extra days. The maternity wing, as any hospital administrator will tell you, generally floats a hospital. The almighty dollar is speaking here."

When Peters wrote that letter, the country was embroiled in a seething debate over the health insurance revolution known as managed care, which was pressuring hospitals to send women home within twenty-four hours of a normal vaginal delivery. Some insurers were paying mothers a hundred or two hundred dollars in cash to leave within a day of giving birth. The first few days after birth, however, are critical for the health of the mother and baby. Should a newborn have difficulty breast-feeding, it quickly can become dehydrated, and need immediate medical help. As well, many newborns suffer from jaundice, which might not be detected until the third day of life. Reports of women fainting and newborns suffering serious complications shortly after discharge elicited a national outcry over "drive-through deliveries."

One of the most publicized cases occurred in May 1995, when Michelina Alanna Bauman was sent home from a New

Jersey hospital twenty-eight hours after she was born. She died the next day of a bacterial infection that her family believes would have been detected, and even eradicated, if she had been kept in the hospital another day. As her parents mourned, the baby's great-uncle, Dominick Ruggiero Jr., a retired bus driver, turned her death into a highly publicized battle against insurance plans. He lobbied the state's governor, Christine Todd Whitman, as well as First Lady Hillary Rodham Clinton, to change the practice. Within a month, Whitman—mother of two, one by cesarean—signed legislation requiring insurers to pay for a second day's stay for vaginal births and four days for cesareans. Other states raced to pass similar laws, and by 1998 federal legislation was in place.

Despite the public outcry and change in laws, there was never any hard evidence that, in the vast majority of cases, discharge within a day was harmful. Researchers pored over the records of twenty thousand mother-baby pairs between 1990 and 1998 and reported that the rate of emergency room visits and hospital readmissions for newborns remained constant, regardless of whether mothers stayed twenty-four or forty-eight hours in the hospital. Still, insurers did not to try to reverse hospital policy because they realized they could front-load most of their maternity charges on the first day of hospitalization. That extra day of care cost them minimally, not worth the public relations nightmare.

ROOMING-IN

The lying-in period in hospitals used to be a solitary time. Before the late twentieth century, maternity wards were actually promoted as places where women could give birth free of the burden of caring for their households; babies did not room with their mothers. They were kept in separate nurseries under policies that were so strict that even those mothers who desperately wanted to remain with their babies rarely could.

At the time, hospitals were afraid that newborns would catch infections from their mothers or the other women sharing the room (in the 1920s and '30s, some cramped hospitals still had women sharing beds). Concerns about infection were so great that staffs followed intricate antisepsis routines that included washing the mother's perineum with Lysol every four hours and cleaning her nipples with a boric acid solution before and after each feeding. Boston Lying-In built its first nursery in 1922 after a baby caught diphtheria from another mother's chronic ear discharge.

The nurseries, however, did not prevent infection. They incubated impetigo, diarrhea, and respiratory illnesses. The germs spread so quickly that some hospitals began to see that babies were better off with their mothers and insisted the two stay together. The situation was reversed at rapid speed, often with unnecessary rigidity.

The concept of "rooming-in"—a term coined by Yale child psychologists Arnold Gesell and Frances L. Ilg in 1943—was introduced during the World War II era, when hospital crowding forced the facilities to have mothers and babies room together. Now that antibiotics had arrived, doctors no longer feared infectious outbreaks. Meanwhile, Freudian psychology had given rise to theories that criminal behavior and psychiatric disorders were caused by poor mother-child relationships, relationships that began the first day of life. If hospitals could help a mother meet her child's needs immediately, the world would stop creating the likes of Hitler, whose reign of terror loomed large in the postwar years. Such a change in parenting theory pushed women to become more responsive to their babies' cries.

Still, the rooming-in concept was slow to spread. As late as 1958, a survey of three thousand U.S. hospitals found that only three hundred allowed mother and child to remain together. By the 1960s, nursing shortages had abated, as had the birth rate, but babies were still being sent to nurseries. Psychologists made it clear that mothers alone did not shape a child's personality or

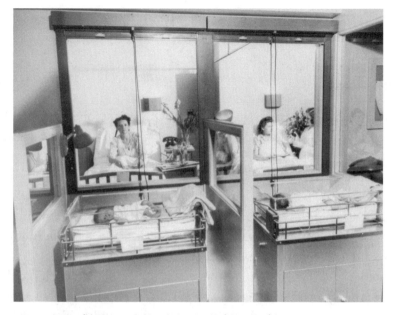

At George Washington University Hospital in Washington, D.C., postpartum recovery rooms overlooked the nursery, circa the 1940s. (Courtesy the National Library of Medicine)

psyche. And more than a decade after the atomic bomb made some worry about technology's effects on humans, space travel renewed public interest and trust in science, which included the standardized environment of the nursery. In 1963, a maternity wing at the Baptist Memorial Hospital in Memphis, Tennessee, even installed closed-circuit cameras, so mothers could watch their infants from their postpartum beds.

Of course, not all mothers were comfortable being separated from their babies. One desperate woman told the *New York Times* in 1950 that she paid the hospital cleaning lady to report on how her baby was doing in the nursery. In 1975, a Houston mother told the newspaper that she was stunned to visit friends in the hospital "and see them looking at their babies in the nursery behind the window. I can't believe that grown people let this happen to them."

She was not alone in questioning the logic of nurseries.

BONDING

Marshall Klaus, the American doctor who championed the use of doulas, was a young respiratory physiologist and neonatologist in the 1960s. Working at a Stanford preemie nursery, he came across a surprising case. A mother, who had tried for five years to become pregnant, delivered a 4-pound baby about five weeks early. The child was blue and needed oxygen. It was sent to the special nursery, which the mother was not allowed to enter. The newborn was put on a respirator initially but rapidly improved. Klaus told the mother that the baby merely needed to gain weight, which it did, reaching 5.5 pounds several weeks later. When the mother took the baby home, she had difficulty feeding it and held the child tentatively, as if it were a stranger.

"Maybe if the mother [had been] able to touch the baby and hold the baby and care for the baby right away, she would have appreciated that the baby was now well," Klaus recalled in an interview. "That set me on the path of learning when the mother becomes bonded to the baby."

In 1967 Klaus joined forces with John Kennell, then a professor of pediatrics at Case Western Reserve University School of Medicine in Cleveland, to look at whether mothers of preemies handled their babies differently than those with full-term infants. They found that preemie mothers were very hands-off during the pediatric office visits, even reading *Life* magazine while Dr. Klaus inspected the baby. It was as if the preemie mothers were afraid they would hurt their infants, even though the babies were now healthy. The full-term mothers, by contrast, were much more involved during the exams, standing next to Dr. Klaus, handing him diapers, soothing the newborns.

Klaus's hunch appears to have been correct. The lack of immediate contact between mothers and preemies had long-term, deleterious implications. Contact is good for babies—and their parents—right from the beginning. And it improves not just their relationship. Allowing time to bond helps increase childhood IQ scores, keeps families intact, and reduces the likelihood of child abuse, he says.

The doctors' groundbreaking research helped convince hospitals to change their nursery practices, not just for preemies and those babies who needed intensive care, but for all newborns. In 1970, the American Medical Association decided that even a ten-minute bonding period immediately after birth should be standard in U.S. hospitals. Today, most hospitals request mothers to room-in full-time with their newborns.

So how to facilitate bonding? Immediate skin-to-skin contact acts as a primer for it, minimizing newborn crying and piquing the baby's interest in nursing. Breast-feeding triggers a powerful hormonal cocktail beneficial to both parties. The mother and baby experience a surge of oxytocin, which increases the woman's and probably the baby's pain threshold—and helps the uterus contract. Oxytocin also calms them and helps the baby absorb needed nutrients.

Roman philosophers and moralists did not need such scientific evidence to tell them that breast-feeding led to bonding. They were against wet nursing because they saw how attached infants became to these women who were not their mothers. Furthermore, postpartum separation among most mammal species often leads to a mother rejecting its young. Of course, the vast majority of women would never choose to give up a baby just because they were separated, but in the rare case that a mother was predisposed to giving up a child, keeping them apart early could be a deciding factor.

In 1990, UNICEF, in an attempt to boost breast-feeding

around the world, issued a ten-point program called the "Baby-Friendly Initiative," recommending that hospitals close their nurseries and stop offering bottles and pacifiers. The program had remarkable success—but not just for breast-feeding. In countries as diverse as Russia, Thailand, and Costa Rica, where infant abandonment was high in hospitals, keeping mothers and babies together helped them bond. In one Thai hospital, where thirty-three out of every ten thousand newborns were given up by their mothers, the figure dropped to one out of ten thousand by 1991.

LEBOYER BABY BATHS

Those first days for any newborn are a shock to its system. Around the world, many cultures have tried to ease the infant's adjustment from the womb to the outside world.

In the fourteenth century, an English monk named Bartholomew said babies should enter the world in a room that is warm, quiet, and dark, much like the womb. On Easter Island, natives would expose their newborns to the harshness of daylight only gradually, a practice they thought resulted in excellent night vision. And in the 1930s, Maria Montessori, the Italian woman who revolutionized early education for children, wrote that a newborn "arrives in the adult world with delicate eyes which have never seen daylight and ears which have never known noise. His body, hitherto unbruised, is now exposed to rough contact with the soulless hands of an adult who disregards that delicacy which should be respected." Montessori lived in a time when newborns were held upside down by their feet and spanked in an effort to make sure their lungs were cleared and they could breathe. Proof was in the cry.

The practice of spanking wasn't to change until the 1970s, when French obstetrician Frederick Leboyer popularized a new theory. Leboyer believed that newborns were acutely sensitive, not just to the new reality of life disconnected from the umbilical cord, but to the birth process itself. Birth, he said, is "the torture of an innocent."

"That tragic expression, those tight-shut eyes, those twitching eyebrows," Leboyer wrote, sounding more like a poet than a doctor, in his radical and groundbreaking book *Birth without Violence,* first published in France in 1974. "That howling mouth, that squirming head trying desperately to find refuge. . . . Those hands stretching out to us, imploring, begging, then retreating to shield the face—that gesture of dread. Those furiously kicking feet, those arms that suddenly pull downward to protect the stomach. The flesh that is one great shudder. This baby is not speaking? Every inch of the body is crying out: 'Don't touch me!' And at the same time pleading: 'Don't leave me! Help me!' Has there ever been a more heartrending appeal?"

The book, a best seller in France, and later published around the world, recommended having the lights dimmed and the room in near silence. But in Leboyer's initial tests, mothers found the quiet so frightening they assumed something was terribly wrong.

"My baby's dead!" a mother would shout.

"Your child's doing wonderfully," Leboyer would tell her quietly before shushing her, which would upset her even more. "Dead! My baby's dead!"

He would point to the child on her belly and whisper, "Dead children are completely still. Feel your baby moving. Feel how happy he is!"

Women were so conditioned to listen for their baby's cry that the silence seemed like torture.

Leboyer also recommended some postpartum practices that seemed radical at the time. He said doctors should cut the umbilical cord only after it stopped pulsing (usually between three and six minutes postpartum). He, or the mother, would gently massage the baby as it lay skin to skin on her belly. And because

Leboyer believed the last thing newborns wanted was to be plunked down on a cold metal scale, he advocated giving them immediate warm baths.

"For the baby has emerged from water, the maternal waters that have carried it, caressed and cradled it," Leboyer wrote. "As the baby sinks down [into the bath], it becomes weightless, and is set free of the body that is overwhelming it—this body with all its burden of harsh new sensation. . . . Its surprises, its joy are boundless." Slowly, he said, the infant should be lifted out of the water and then gently dipped back in again, a sort of practice run for the bath's conclusion. The child should then be wrapped in layers of cotton and wool but with its head and hands free to move. "The quiet, newborn baby radiates the most intense peace," Leboyer says at the end of the book. "Completely awake, supremely alert, this baby glows."

What would you rather have? A newborn shrieking itself purple or a child as heavenly as the one described above? Of course, mothers in the 1970s opted for the latter, demanding Leboyer baths alongside their hospital beds. Doctors generally were opposed to the baths, seeing them as a frivolous nuisance as well as a potential hazard: Working with water in a darkened room could be slippery. "I don't see any logic or sense" to the baths, Dr. Patricia Burkhardt, the manager of the nurse-midwifery department at Columbia-Presbyterian, said in 1989, when women were still requesting the Leboyer method and hospitals were still obliging.

Nurses also hated the method because they had to fill the tubs.

"We nurses had suspicions about that latest gimmick in a decade full of gimmicks, but in the interest of keeping new mothers happy, we tried to accommodate them. We developed a system that worked sort of okay, some of the time, for some of the babies," wrote Peggy Vincent in her 2002 book *Baby Catcher: Chronicles of a Modern Midwife*. "We filled a seamless Plexiglas crib at the scrub sink with about four gallons of water, which was as much as we could lift without risking back injuries, and replaced it on its wheeled metal cart. Then we added more water to adjust the temperature just before pushing the cart into the delivery room. Something always seemed amiss—too hot, too cold, too shallow, too deep. Of course, no one can predict the exact time of a baby's birth. While we waited, the water cooled to the point that it was not a pleasant experience for the baby when we lowered them into the tub, and the babies often screamed until we took them out."

But Leboyer baths infiltrated popular culture. R. D. Laing, a Scottish psychoanalyst, provided the on- and off-screen commentary for a powerful one-hour documentary film in 1978 called *Birth, with R. D. Laing*, which showed the gut-wrenching standard hospital treatment of newborns. The film, shot in New Zealand, aired first in the UK and then the United States, and further stirred the debate about newborn care. When writer Nora Ephron was pregnant in the late 1970s, she said her Lamaze teacher pushed the Leboyer method. Four days after witnessing thirty African babies receive the baths, the teacher saw that the infants seemed to have better muscle control and were less tense than their American counterparts.

"Don't tell me about four days," Ephron wrote. "Tell me about college entrance examinations." When someone in Ephron's Lamaze class asked what she should do if the doctor refused to deliver by the Leboyer method, the teacher told the class, "If you can't have Leboyer, it's your kid's karma."

Soon enough, though, studies began debunking any real benefits of the bath. A 1980 Canadian study in the *New England Journal of Medicine* found that minute-by-minute observations showed no significant differences between infants who were given the baths and those who weren't.

Leboyer baths were a passing fad. But two other longer lasting ideas emerged from Leboyer's theories. First, as a matter of standard practice, obstetricians no longer hold newborns by the ankles and spank them. They are now handled gently, often placed skin to skin on their mother's belly, and the lights are often kept dim, except in the operating room.

BREAST-FEEDING

Handling a newborn gently, placing the child immediately in its mother's arms—such changes in maternity care were suddenly facilitating the reemergence of another natural element of birth: breast-feeding.

In the moments after delivery, most babies, if placed on their mother's bellies, will actually shinny up toward the breast and try to latch on. But they won't find milk. Not yet. Before the breasts become engorged, a few days postpartum, colostrum is all a mother has to offer her newborn. Although we now know the substance helps babies purge meconium and boosts their immunity, colostrum has been shunned since ancient times. The creamy yellow goop does not look like milk, and women in many cultures have refused to feed such a foul-looking thing to their offspring. Throughout Nepal and much of South Asia, women considered colostrum as disgusting as pus. Hindus did not allow mothers to nurse for the first few days, until a priest approved it, because the fluid was considered unfit. That's still the case in many preindustrialized societies.

Some societies believed that even once a woman's milk had come in, the mother should not breast-feed when she's bleeding, which can last, perfectly normally, for weeks postpartum. In ancient Greece, Soranus told mothers to wait three weeks after birth, when she not only would have "real" milk but would feel up to the task of suckling. In the seventeenth century, some European mothers withheld breast-feeding for the first month, sending the baby to suckle on a wet nurse or domesticated animal. In France, foundling hospitals kept goats on the premises so newborns could suck directly from them, the animals straddling the cradles.

These practices could have grave consequences. When a newborn sucks on its mother, it stimulates the production of milk and oxytocin; without regular sucking, a woman's milk dries up. (It's possible but not easy to start up again.) So if a mother couldn't breast-feed, she would have to either commit the baby to a wet nurse or feed the newborn with animal milk or some other substance, such as honey or sugar water. In the days before sterilization or formula, feeding a newborn anything but breast milk directly could be lethal, especially if the baby had not received the early immunities that colostrum provided. Medical texts from the 1500s said the most common newborn ailment was "gripes" or bowel looseness, a problem that could lead to fatal dehydration but could go away if and when a baby started breast-feeding.

Throughout history, women have fed animal milk to babies using spouted clay jugs, linen, horns, and pickled cow nipples. Archaeologists have found evidence of infant feeding vessels in grave sites dating back to 4000 BC. Yet, these containers inevitably harbored deadly germs. At the Dublin Foundling Hospital, of ten thousand hand-fed infants between 1775 and 1796, only forty-five survived infancy, an astounding mortality rate of 99.6 percent.

People knew that the indirect feeding of any milk could kill a newborn, although they did not know why. In the south of France, one monsignor was so alarmed by high infant mortality rates that he offered bounties to mothers who breast-fed for the first year, a successful program that reduced deaths by 33 percent.

Allowing the child to suck directly from a domesticated animal, such as a cow or goat, had other complications. The milk from those animals can be difficult if not impossible for some newborns to digest. Ancient Greeks and Romans found the idea of drinking the milk of another species disgusting. Greeks referred to barbarians as *galaktopotes*, or dairy drinkers. In Italy, early medical writers told mothers that if they let their baby drink from animals, the child would always look "stupid and vacant and not right in the head."

When mothers didn't breast-feed, it wasn't just bad for their babies; it had consequences for mothers, as well. With their milk stagnating, women were more susceptible to potentially fatal breast infections, which, in the seventeenth and eighteenth centuries, were as dreaded as puerperal fever. Around 1750, England's William Hunter (Smellie's old friend) tried reducing the death rate at a lying-in hospital by forcing mothers to breast-feed their babies immediately, rather than wait the customary three to four days postpartum. Milk fever went away, and newborns fared much better, too. For those who did nurse their babies within the first week, women still drew out the colostrum beforehand using a cupping glass, an older "lusty" child, or even a puppy.

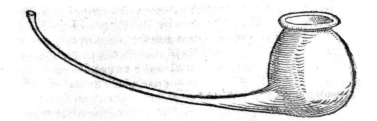

German woodcut, circa 1545, of a sucking glass, an early breast pump. (Courtesy the Wellcome Library)

Of course, some women could not breast-feed. The baby might have had a cleft palate that made sucking difficult. The mother might have been ill, on the verge of death, or forced to work. She might have had inverted nipples, a common affliction from wearing tightly laced dresses and corsets beginning in girlhood. Some might have had no nipples at all, the consequence of ulcerations or the long-term nursing of toothy children. The logical thing in those situations was to have the baby suck from another lactating woman—a wet nurse. In Africa, grandmothers sometimes still do this for the tribe; there have been reports of women lactating into their eighties.

Formalized wet nursing dates back to the Pharaonic era, when royal babies were almost always suckled by someone other than its mother. If a wet nurse's own child shared the breast with an unrelated baby, the children were called milk-sisters or milk-brothers. In ancient Mesopotamia, legal contracts safeguarded such feeding arrangements for as long as two years. Ancient Greeks and Romans used slaves as wet nurses.

Choosing a wet nurse was not a minor task. In India, a wet nurse had to come from the same caste as the child she was feeding; the nurse's own children had to be alive; and her nipples had to be perfect. Many cultures believed that a nurse's personal attributes, even her moral character, her height, or her hair color could be passed to the baby through the milk. The tyrant emperor Caligula, for example, was supposedly nursed by a bloodthirsty woman. And in the pre–Civil War American South, many black nannies nursed white children (though some white families refused black wet nurses out of fear their offspring would grow up talking and acting like slaves).

There are several reasons—beyond necessity—that some women chose not to breast-feed their own. Galen, in the second century, said semen in a woman's body soured her breast milk, a belief that persisted until the Middle Ages, when children were generally weaned around two years of age. Given that notion, one could see why some husbands may have pressured their wives to give up nursing—or implored them never to start. The Catholic Church, until the eighteenth century, encouraged the use of wet nurses so that a wife could pay her husband "his conjugal due." (Of course, then the wet nurse was not to have sex with *her* husband.) The church's views helped wet nursing become embedded in predominantly Catholic France, where the state began controlling the practice as early as the thirteenth century. Of the twenty-one thousand babies born in Paris in 1780, only about one thousand were nursed by their own mothers. Because wet nurses were in such demand, French law mandated that women could not take on new infants until their own babies were nine months old.

In Protestant England and its colonies, wet nurses were more common among the very poor (whose babies ended up in foundling hospitals) and the very rich (who shopped for wet nurses among the lactating destitutes freshly delivered in lying-in hospitals). The upper class would often send their babies to live with the nurse in the country—hence, the term *farmed out*—and parental visits could be separated by months. It's possible that one reason wealthy women did not breast-feed is they knew it decreased their chances of becoming pregnant again. Having large families was fashionable for upper-class European women, whose status grew with every arranged marriage of their children. Poor women, who could not afford to care for throngs of their own children, benefited from the income wet nursing provided, as well as its de facto birth control.

For the poor, wet nursing was actually a desirable profession, usually paying more than any other work a woman might have. These women worked hard to maintain their supply of milk. In the fourteenth and fifteenth centuries, German wet nurses were told to eat powdered earthworms and massage their breasts with the ashes of burnt owls. Egyptians used spells, potions, and incantations to increase their milk supply. Pacific Islanders suckled piglets to keep their milk flowing between jobs.

Some women, though, are just natural producers, and in many countries there is an outlet for their overabundance and generosity: milk banks. The first human milk bank was established in Vienna in 1909, followed by two others, in Boston and Germany, in 1919. These banks refrigerated and dispensed donated milk for sick, orphaned, premature, and multiple-birth babies. By the 1980s, the AIDS crisis had forced the closure of many milk banks out of concern for contaminated milk. But rigid screening guidelines were later established. Today, frozen donor milk is sent to the bank, thawed, pasteurized, tested, refrozen, and shipped overnight to hospitals or homes. As more studies show how unique breast milk is, the number of banks has rebounded. There are about a dozen in the United States and Canada. Although most milk banks rely on charity "donations," in some countries, such as Sweden and Denmark, women have received more than twenty dollars per liter, tax free, for sending their breast milk to a bank.

Newborns over the centuries have been fed lots of other things besides breast milk: water, honey, and pap, which is mashed food. In 1867, a German chemist named Liebig devised a new formula of cow's milk, flour, potassium bicarbonate, and malt. Although the public, increasingly afraid of syphilis being transmitted through infected sores, was ready to replace wet nursing and direct animal feeding, they did not seem that impressed with his "formula," either. For one thing, it was difficult to prepare. However, that same year, Henri Nestlé, who had been working for some time to invent a replacement for a mother's nourishment, devised a mix of milk and flour that he tested on a gravely ill infant who took to the formula. Widespread news of the baby's rebound caused sales of Nestlé's formula to soar.

Although infant formula initially was for feeding orphans and sick children, by the early twentieth century manufacturers had begun to present the product as an option for all newborns. Their marketing campaigns coincided with the increase in the number of babies in hospital nurseries. Formula makers showed hospitals how the product could benefit everyone, and doctors accepted free samples in exchange for lavish gifts and research grants. Some companies even employed "milk nurses"—paid on commission—who would visit mothers in hospitals to sell formula.

Once mothers were home, however, inadequate refrigeration, bad water, and lack of proper bottle sterilization caused germs to breed in the formula, and in warm weather babies frequently developed "summer complaint," potentially fatal diarrhea caused by the contamination. The ignorance and confusion surrounding bottle preparation spurred Nathan Straus, owner of Macy's department store in New York, to give away pasteurized milk to poor children at philanthropic "stations," a concept that had also taken hold in Europe, where weekly infant weigh-ins were part of the exchange. In New York, mothers who were not going to breast-feed were lured to the stations by the free milk and then taught how to safely use bottles. These stations, combined with hospital nursery policies, made it possible and even fashionable for women not to breast-feed as the twentieth century progressed. Later, with the industrialization of American foods and women's modern desires to free themselves of domesticated duties, even more mothers were driven to use formula.

By 1956, the year Mary White convened the first meeting of the breast-feeding advocacy group La Leche League in her Illinois home, only 20 percent of American mothers were breast-feeding. (The group chose the name—*la leche* means milk in Spanish—because it was considered impolite to utter the words *breast-feeding* and *pregnancy*.) In 1957, La Leche League invited Grantly Dick-Read to speak to a packed house at a local high school, where he advocated breast-feeding as part of natural childbirth. The concept gained momentum and by 1972, breast-feeding rates in the United States had begun to rise and would continue to climb an average of 3 percent a year through the end of that decade.

At the same time, however, formula companies were redirecting their advertising campaigns to the undeveloped world. Although some doctors endorsed formula as a way to fight malnutrition, sterilizing bottles properly proved impossible for people who had no sanitary water or little fuel for boiling water. As missionaries and public health workers began to see bottle-fed infants dying in alarming numbers in places such as Nigeria, they became concerned. In 1974, a British charity, The War on Want, published *The Baby Killer,* a report whose cover featured a drawing of a malnourished black baby who was crying and crammed inside a bottle. The treatise, which exposed how formula companies tried to capture their markets, triggered a boycott of Nestlé products. Meanwhile, the World Health Organization called for a review of formula sales practices, which resulted in a code of ethics for companies to follow. Yet one year later, a documentary film entitled *Bottle Babies* showed mothers in Kenya still mixing filthy water with powdered food, and infant graves marked with prized formula cans.

With further scientific evidence emerging that the breast was best, a generation of American women who had been bottle fed themselves was wising up to how formula companies had infiltrated the market. Today, 70 percent of new American mothers are breast-feeding, encouraged by a new breed of helpers: lactation consultants. Unlike the "milk nurses" of yore, these professionals teach mothers everything from how to get a baby to latch on to the breast, to how to promote her own milk production.

BABY BLUES

The hormonal changes during and immediately after birth often are gloriously beneficial. Nature's cocktail of oxytocin, progesterone, and endorphins help a woman love, nurture, and feed her baby. The hormones also fight off pain, prevent severe bleeding, and even bestow her with a warm glow.

Yet, profound hormonal shifts about a day after delivery can work against some women. Progesterone and estrogen, which helped sustain the pregnancy, plummet to levels not experienced before conception, and many women feel weepy, irritable, and moody for at least a couple of weeks postpartum. For a small group, this can develop into something more serious than the "baby blues." Ten to 20 percent of women suffer from serious postpartum depression; they show little interest in the newborn and neglect their own daily routines such as eating or sleeping. Another fraction of a percent develop postpartum psychosis, which can include hallucinations and suicidal or homicidal actions.

Probably the most famous case of postpartum psychosis is that of Andrea Yates, a Texas woman who, in 2001, drowned her five children—including a six-month-old—in a bathtub. Prosecutors called for the death penalty, arguing that as long as she could distinguish between right and wrong, having postpartum psychosis is no excuse for murder. Because Yates testified that she knew it was a crime to kill her children, a jury convicted her of capital murders in 2002, triggering debate about whether the standard for mental illness was too rigid and whether the courts understood the nature of postpartum mental illness. But an appeals court overturned that conviction due to erroneous testimony, and after a new trial in 2006, a jury found her not guilty by reason of insanity. Rather than send her to prison for life, the judge committed her to a locked mental hospital until she is deemed no longer a threat. In response to the second verdict, legal experts said that, in the four years since the Yates case had been in court, the American public had become more understanding—even forgiving—of postpartum depression. Perhaps that is the only good to emerge from such a tragedy.

In more than two dozen countries, including Great Britain, Canada, and Australia, postpartum depression can be used as a legal defense if a mother kills her child in its first year of life. The most she can face is a manslaughter charge, often with probation and counseling. The United States does not have this type of national legislation, and laws vary so much among states that a mother could be convicted of anything from unlawful disposal of a corpse (a misdemeanor with probation) to first-degree murder (a felony with life in prison, perhaps even punishable by death depending on the jurisdiction).

Although we hear more about postpartum depression these days through sensational stories—a new mother jumping off a bridge or driving her children into a lake—it is an ancient problem. And it has been misunderstood for nearly as long. Two thousand years ago Hippocrates believed new mothers went mad because their breast milk was diverted to their brains. Not until the 1960s and '70s, when the culture was more willing to talk about mental illness, as well as the emotional upheaval of becoming parents, did postpartum depression begin to draw serious attention. The *New York Times* archives shows that the first mention of "postpartum depression" in that paper was in 1968, in an article that publicized studies that tracked weepy suburban housewives in the weeks after delivery. As new headlines and new research began to stockpile, some even wondered if the emotional upset was a self-made phenomenon, perpetuated by new parents under pressure to balance work and home, without the help of extended family.

But a 1988 study shattered that notion, finding that in Uganda, although mothers had more elaborate support networks and postpartum rituals than their counterparts in Scotland, 10 percent of the African women developed depression, compared with about 13 percent in Scotland. Postpartum depression was beginning to be seen as a universal affliction. More recently, scientists have begun researching how post-pregnancy endocrinology, including lower serotonin levels, could trigger the illness. With the public's consciousness raised, the illness could then slip into the realm of pop culture.

In the spring of 2005, actor Brooke Shields disclosed in a memoir that she had developed postpartum depression after the birth of her first child and was prescribed Paxil, a drug her doctor said would be safe to take while breast-feeding. "I was feeling so bad that I found it hard to believe that a tiny pink pill could lift the black cloud," she wrote in *Down Came the Rain*. She began to feel better and then quit the drug cold. A few days later she fantasized about driving into a wall, with the baby in the car. She promptly went back on the drug.

As if the book weren't enough to get people talking about it, fellow celebrity Tom Cruise, a member of the Church of Scientology —which does not believe in psychiatric medicine—publicly criticized Shields for taking the antidepressants. In a rambling interview on the *Today* show, host Matt Lauer pressed him about his remarks. Cruise said psychiatry is a "pseudoscience," that drugs "mask the problem," and that "there is no such thing as a chemical imbalance in a body."

Shields fired back with an opinion piece for the *New York Times* explaining that a woman's levels of estrogen and progesterone greatly increase during pregnancy and that, in the first twenty-four hours after childbirth those hormone levels plunge, sometimes triggering restlessness and irritability, sadness, and hopelessness. "If any good can come of Mr. Cruise's ridiculous rant, let's hope that it gives much-needed attention to a serious disease. Perhaps now is the time to call on doctors, particularly obstetricians and pediatricians, to screen for postpartum depression," she wrote. "After all, during the first three months after childbirth, you see a pediatrician at least three times." Shields's suggestion for such screening should not be dismissed.

After thousands of years of misunderstanding postpartum depression, ignoring its symptoms, or being shocked by its ramifications, the problem needs attention, whether from a baby doctor or two celebrities having a spat in the national spotlight.

IN THE END

THROUGHOUT THE PROCESS of writing this book, whenever people heard about its subject, they invariably said something like, "Oh, you're writing about how women used to die?" I'd get this remark at a party or at the playground. I'd stammer, "Well, yes and no" and then try to explain further, although that was never easy to do while hors d'oeuvres were being passed or kids were screaming. So I will attempt a clear response here.

The prospect of death in childbirth has always loomed large —even though women were just as likely to die from an infected finger, a persistent cough, or a disease. On Panape, a small island in the South Pacific, when a woman was about six months pregnant, she and her husband would visit her parents and other relatives for a feast called *kamweng kasapw*. This was not a celebration of impending motherhood. It was a send-off, in case she died giving birth. In Chad, a local proverb says that a pregnant woman has one foot in the grave. In seventeenth-century America, the only publication of any obstetrical significance was a little book called *A Present to Be Given to Teeming Women by Their Husbands or Friends Containing Scripture-Directions for Women with Child, How to Prepare for the Hour of [Travail]*. The book told pregnant women to pray, repent, read scripture, and prepare for death. And in the American West, pioneer women made out their wills before going into labor. So how common has death been in childbirth throughout time?

The diary of the Reverend Ezra Stiles, president of Yale College in the late eighteenth century, noted that between 1760 and 1764 there were ten maternal deaths in Newport, Rhode Island, a rate of one-half of 1 percent. These were probably fairly pure births, in an age of simple midwifery, few tools, and no anesthesia. In natural and historical terms, a half of 1 percent is not a lot. Of course, no one would want to be one of the women who died, or her offspring.

In the nineteenth century, when most women around the world still gave birth at home, maternal mortality was fairly constant at about 1 percent. While that number seems egregiously high today, tuberculosis killed more women of childbearing age than birth did. Outside of big cities, maternal mortality was slightly lower.

However—and this is where my questioner would usually look for a fresh glass of wine or make her way toward the sandbox —by the early 1900s, maternal mortality rates were increasing sharply, especially in urban areas. Disease, decreasing numbers of midwives, and more meddlesome practices were introducing new troubles in childbirth. Government and charities sprang into action. Prenatal clinics, a brand-new concept, opened in Edinburgh, Boston, and Sydney. But death rates continued to rise.

By 1932, with midwifery in decline and the number of hospitals growing, maternal mortality in New York City had risen to alarming levels. Excluding deaths from ectopic pregnancies—in which the gestation occurs outside the uterus—and abortions, 4.5 percent of women who delivered in hospitals died after what should have been a normal delivery, compared to 1.6 percent of those who delivered at home with a midwife. And at least half of the deaths were preventable, according to a landmark report by the New York Academy of Medicine.

"Frequently the operation chosen was the wrong one," the report said. "Often it was undertaken at an improper time. Manifestly obstructed labors were allowed to continue when it should have been clear that delivery could not be effected from below. Trial labors were frequently too greatly prolonged." The report also noted that the hospitals had bad equipment and poor facilities, lacked supervision, and allowed junior residents to handle complicated operations. It concluded by saying, "The relative safety of delivery at home should be emphasized."

Another report, on maternal mortality in Boston, found that between 1933 and 1935, 0.6 percent of mothers and 2 percent of babies were dying in birth. Women were killed by cesareans, "careless anesthesia," ectopic pregnancy, hemorrhage, badly administered pituitrin (an early Pitocin), toxemia, and air embolism in an intravenous drip. But the two greatest killers, the report concluded, were infection and botched abortions. "Little need be said about the preventability of these deaths," the authors, all doctors, wrote.

Fortunately, almost every decade since then, maternal mortality rates in developed countries have decreased. In the 1930s, sulfa drugs began fighting infections, every year saving tens of thousands of women who would otherwise have died of puerperal sepsis or bungled abortions. In the 1940s, doctors began treating hemorrhages with replenishing transfusions and drugs such as ergometrine and oxytocin, which helped the uterus contract and stop excessive bleeding. Postwar policies of getting mothers out of bed soon after birth lowered the number of fatal blood clots, and better anesthesia made the likelihood of a related death almost zero. Throughout the 1950s, women's health and nutrition generally improved. By the 1960s, abortion had established itself as the most common cause of maternal death and remained so until Britain and the United States legalized it.

Yet despite all the advancements available today—rubber gloves, safer cesareans, blood pressure monitoring, diagnostic ultrasound, and antibiotics, to name a few—500,000 women (that's one every minute) die in childbirth. Ninety-nine percent of them live in the developing world. Black women, especially those in sub-Saharan Africa, are the most likely to perish, while women from the whitest cultures, such as Sweden and Austria, are the least likely. Americans may feel smugly safe, but twenty-five countries —including Qatar and Slovakia—have better records when it comes to mothers surviving birth, according to the World Health Organization (WHO).

Today, according to WHO, 25 percent of maternal deaths are from hemorrhage, 15 percent from infection, 13 percent from unsafe abortions, 12 percent from eclampsia, and 8 percent from obstructed labor, a category that includes placenta previa.

Yet for all the perils a woman might face, birth is more than one hundred times deadlier for the baby. It has always been this way. Attitudes about helping newborns survive began to change in the nineteenth century, a shift that historians have attributed, in part, to the rise in democracy after the French and American revolutions, an awakening to humanitarianism, and the increasing industrialization that demanded larger populations to work in factories.

In France in the late nineteenth century, 30 percent of newborns weighed less than 5 pounds, 9 ounces, at birth, and only 20 percent lived to be a year old. In 1880, amid heightened concern about the country's fragile population, obstetrician E. S. Tarnier invented the incubator, which he modeled after the warming devices a zookeeper in Paris had devised for hatching chickens. Tarnier named the wooden incubator a *couveuse*, which translates as "brooding hen." (The public was fascinated with the idea of seeing tiny babies living in ovens, and the newborns and their incubators became a bizarre hit at the World Exposition in Berlin in 1896, outshining the nearby Congo Village and Tyrolean Yodelers.) Before the incubators were invented, premature infants were wrapped in sheepskin, placed in jars of feathers, set in cots in front of a fire, or placed on hot water bottles to keep them warm. In 1898, Joseph B. DeLee, the prophylactic forceps operator, established America's first premature infant incubator station, in Chicago. That same year, two Paris hospitals developed "weakling" departments, precursors to neonatal intensive care units.

Other developments were also helping fragile infants survive. In 1912, New York launched a campaign that sent nurses to visit new mothers at home; the rate of newborn deaths dropped. By 1950, better overall health, prenatal care, strident attitudes about the importance of sterility for infant feeding, and the rise in cesarean safety for the most difficult cases, all contributed to a dramatic decline in fatalities.

In 2001, American infant mortality was less than 1 percent. Since then, that figure has increased slightly, mostly because more babies are being born prematurely to older women and women carrying multiples. In many cases, science had helped conceive these children and kept them in the womb but could not guarantee them life. (Prematurity has replaced birth defects as the most common reason babies die. More than 400,000 children annually are now born too early in America, an all-time high.)

Rituals for coping with the loss of a child have been rich and varied throughout time. But when death moved to the hospitals, it disconnected people from the loss of life, as their stillborns were whisked away before parents could see them. Research beginning in the 1940s, however, found that it was deeply important for the bereaved to express grief, something hospitals were not facilitating.

"When I started to cry in the hospital, they wanted to give me a tranquilizer. I would say, 'Gee, if I could just cry, maybe I would get it out of my system,'" said a woman quoted by Marshall Klaus, bonding expert, in his 1976 book. "If mourning is impeded and not allowed to run its course," he said, "pathological grief can result."

Today hospitals encourage physical contact and a chance for families to say hello and good-bye all at once. In the last five years, maternity facilities have begun providing bereavement kits, which include a book on healing and a memory envelope to keep a lock of hair, a hospital bracelet, or a footprint.

Mercifully, death, at least in this part of the world, is not something the vast majority of pregnant women fear anymore— for themselves or their babies. Instead of writing wills during the gestational months, we luxuriate in choosing baby names, sorting through the menu of labor and delivery options, and devising birth plans with the help of Web sites that encourage non-bossy language such as "I am hoping to protect the perineum." Our quest for perfection, and satisfaction, has moved birth well beyond the giving of new life. It has become an expression of our lives—both an act of self-discovery and an extension of our management skills. Women hire violin duets to play during labor, listen to James Taylor on their iPods during cesareans, make placenta prints (suitable for framing) while lying-in, and encourage their five-year-olds to catch the baby.

In another century, these birth plans will be perfect time capsules of postmodern maternity, for if there is one thing that writing this book has taught me, it is that birth always reflects the culture in which it happens. In patriarchal societies such as Islamic Bangladesh, conditions are poor, there is rarely help, and many women die. But in Polynesia, where fertility is esteemed, new mothers are pampered and have skilled midwifery help. In Victorian times, upper-class women were encouraged to be frail, and childbirth seemed so unbearable they wanted no part of it, so they slept right through delivery. In the 1940s and 1950s, women—including my grandmother—were tethered to the home and strapped down in the hospital. In the 1970s, the liberation movement awakened women and empowered them to break free; conscious birth in new places became a badge of honor. In the 1990s, as women struggled to maintain balance in their lives, they chose to be part of birth, but without the pain, and so they signed up for epidurals.

And now, as more professional women give birth later in life to fewer children, we can decide in advance how much pain we'll tolerate, where we'd like to give birth, and in what position. We can choose whom we'd like to have with us throughout labor and delivery, be it midwife, doula, obstetrician, father, boyfriend, same-sex partner, egg donor, adoptive parent, child, best friend, coworker—or any combination thereof. The emphasis is on minimizing risk and controlling every aspect of birth—including when it happens. Book a date for induction or cesarean and you can even have the birth announcements printed before the baby arrives. One less unknown having to do with delivery. One more task crossed off the list.

Of course, modern life has also made birth less predictable in some ways. Today's fast-paced mobility has led to babies being born in places as high as 30,000 feet, in an airplane, or below ground, on a train. In 2003, on a morning rush-hour subway car in Boston, a woman quietly delivered a baby, which fell to the floor, sliding among the feet of horrified commuters. The mother, a former nurse who was trying to get to the hospital on time, picked the child up, clutched a handrail, stared out the window as if nothing had happened, and politely refused offers of assistance. Witnesses screamed as the train pulled into the station. The woman exited, but as she bolted for the stairs, the placenta dropped onto the platform. She stuffed the afterbirth in her shoulder bag and kept going before authorities tracked her down to make sure she and the baby were okay.

A more euphoric scene unfolded in 1994 when a woman six months pregnant went into labor on board a TWA flight that had left Kennedy Airport in New York, bound for Orlando.

"Is there a physician on board?" a member of the crew pleaded over the intercom. A flight attendant hurried to clear a row and an internist, headed to Disney World with his wife and three kids, immediately went to the side of the mother-to-be.

"My adrenaline was flowing at a hundred miles an hour," said the man, who had only delivered one baby in his life, many years before. "At first I thought it was false labor. But then she started bleeding. I took another look and saw the head starting to crown, and I said, 'This lady is having this baby right now.'"

As the plane descended for an emergency landing in the Washington area, the infant arrived with the cord wrapped around its neck. The doctor did not think the dark blue child would survive. "I started CPR, massaged the baby's chest with two fingers, and yelled, 'Breathe, baby, breathe.'"

Then a husband-and-wife paramedic team—she had special infant resuscitation training—stepped in to help, calling for a straw to suction mucus from the baby's airway. A flight attendant tore a straw off a juice box stashed in her carry-on. The baby began breathing. A passenger's shoelace tied off the umbilical cord, and the child was swaddled in blue airline blankets.

"It's a boy!" the flight attendant announced. The plane erupted in cheers. All of the 213 passengers gave the mother a standing ovation as she was whisked off board. The four-pound, six-ounce, child's middle name is Dulles, after the Virginia airport where he first touched the earth.

Although we think long and hard about how we want our babies to be born, the decision is often out of our control, even as we waddle up to the hospital admissions desk and tell the staff how we would like the birth to be. As we tick off the options available, we are certain that we have chosen correctly. But have we?

There is no doubt that modern medicine has made astounding advances in the area of birth: infertile women become mothers, sick women deliver healthy babies, and infirm newborns grow into happy kids. But, it must also be said that, for many women, over the years, this supposedly beneficial medical help has often meant isolating babies in nurseries, receiving an unnecessary episiotomy, having a breast dipped in iodine before every feeding —whatever the latest trend. If only we'd known how skeptical we should have been. And should still be. The shot of scopolamine my mother received when I was born was not enough to erase her fear of laboring alone. Those ineffective X-rays she received to check the size of my brother in utero have since been found to cause leukemia. And as for those hee-hee-huuuh breathing exercises she learned, well, my birth instructor told our class not to make such silly noises because they cause hyperventilation.

Yet today, our maternity system is lurching toward its own extreme with defensive practices, labor management checklists, and educated patients who instruct the doctor how they want it to go. It's enough to make you want to turn the clock back—but to when? Lucy's era? Medieval times? The 1970s?

Writing this book certainly gave me the perspective I needed to judge my own experience. But if I could rewind the tape, I doubt there's much I would have changed. Like most women around the world, I am a product of my age, my upbringing, and my culture. I'm not brave enough to have a baby at home—although I respect those who do. I'm too aware of how intensely painful birth can be to cut myself off from the possibility of an epidural, though I admire those who can. I know now that I should have had a midwife—and probably a doula—from the start, but I had too much faith in my anatomy, my husband, and my hospital system to think either was truly necessary. I also realize today that those decisions I made—and those that were made for me—were all part of this great childbirth continuum, which I continue to observe as it unfolds, even in my own family.

In August 2005, I was with my brother's wife, Annmarie, who had stood by the operating table just a few days earlier as her twin sister delivered a breech girl via scheduled cesarean. Annmarie gleefully recalled chatting with her sister, who was numbed from the belly down during the ten-minute procedure. She watched as the obstetrician pulled the girl out by her tiny bottom. Annmarie marveled at the fresh memory, how quick and easy the whole process was, her eyes sparkling as she told the story.

"Annmarie," I asked, already knowing what her answer would be, "when you have a baby, are you asking for a C-section?"

"Yeah!" she said, drawing the word into two syllables, as if I had asked a stupid question. "Who needs labor? With a C-section you know when your baby is going to be born."

Days later, as I was pondering this, my phone rang. It was Julie, my best friend from childhood, calling to tell me that she had delivered her second baby, a son, just a few hours earlier. It all happened so fast, in the middle of the night. There was no time for an epidural.

It hurt. A lot, she said. The baby was over nine pounds.

"But," she whispered, "it was wonderful."

I smiled and felt my eyes water. Finally, I understood that, from country to country, from year to year, the contest between obstetrics and nature will always be in play. Women will forever give birth in many different ways—either by design or through forces out of our control. As for the latter, we can only hope to be pleasantly surprised.

"Congratulations," I whispered to my friend. "You did it."

ACKNOWLEDGMENTS

THE IDEA FOR this book was conceived the day after my son, George, was born, at a time when I was clearly delirious, not comprehending how much work it was to be a mother, let alone write a history. Somehow those things ended up being a delightful combination, working from home with George first on my lap, then crawling around under my chair, then on his own two feet. Time was advancing on the page and before my eyes. Just the other day, when I was typing my final words, he pointed to the screen and said, "Mama's book." It was a bittersweet moment, realizing that he is not a baby anymore and that this other unwieldy creature with a gestation as long as an elephant's was about to be born. George, thank you for being the ultimate inspiration and for showing me miracles can happen every day.

My husband, Anthony Flint, who was working on his own manuscript at the same time, was quite literally always there, down the hall, to offer a suggestion, read a chapter, mix a drink, or manage the house. I am grateful for having such wonderful support and company—and a darn good human thesaurus—during what could have been a very lonely experience.

To my parents, Jack and Gloria Cassidy, thank you for your eternal encouragement, for being my touchstone, and for telling me to write a book long before I ever wanted to or thought I could. I especially appreciate all the wonderful meals you cooked for my hungry household while I was buried in research and for always being interested in what I discovered. You are the best.

My brother, Jake, not only presented me with a freshly built computer specifically for this project but was my own personal IT department. Without his patience and help, I would have had to write it longhand.

Mary Alice Flint, my mother-in-law, painstakingly read early chapters, and her editor's eye helped the work in countless ways. My sister-in-law, Amanda Bower, a force of nature from Down Under, found typos where others were certain there were none.

My grandmother, Genevieve Damaschi, instilled in me early in life that anything is possible—at any age—in spite of adversity. Thank you for being such a wonderful example.

To my agent, Richard Abate at ICM, thank you for your rapid responses, regardless of where you were or what time I was calling. I also want to acknowledge Kate Lee at ICM for smoothly handling all the details, and to my former *Boston Globe* colleague Mitchell Zuckoff for introducing me to Richard.

I especially want to thank Elisabeth Schmitz, my accomplished editor at Grove/Atlantic, for caring not just about the book, but also about the craft. Her careful work, kind words, and high standards were greatly appreciated, and I believe I'll always be a better writer because of what she refused to let me get away with. The rest of the awesome team at Grove/Atlantic, including Dara Hyde and Morgan Entrekin, also deserve special acknowledgment. And to Katie Hall, for that final polish, I owe you considerably.

There are many people to thank at the *Boston Globe,* a second home to me for so many years. First, I am grateful to Caleb Solomon and Martin Baron for graciously granting me time away to write a book on the heels of a prolonged maternity leave. My colleagues Doreen Vigue and Emily Kehe, always great friends, were also phenomenal cheerleaders. Thank you both for your laughter, phone calls, and occasional sushi and champagne. And to Kate Zernike, whose commitment to reading a draft could not even be stopped by Hurricane Katrina whirling overhead, thank you so much.

I am also fortunate to live in a city full of experts, well-stocked libraries, and smart people willing to share their time. Thank you to the obstetric staff at Brigham and Women's Hospital, particularly Dr. William Camann, chief of obstetric anesthesia, whose time and help were invaluable. Now if only he offered epidurals to make writing less painful. I also owe a special thanks to all the mothers at the hospital who welcomed me, a perfect stranger, into their lives at the moment their babies were born. I want to specifically express my gratitude to the Digiammos for being so warm. I would also like to acknowledge obstetricians Toni Golen and especially Alison Steube for answering so many of my questions and for reading a draft. At Boston University, Eugene Declercq and Mary Barger were generous with their time, as were so many others whom I interviewed for this book. And to the wonderful staff at the Cambridge Birth Center, you went out of your way to help me.

Harvard's Countway Library of Medicine has an astonishing rare books collection, which was a deep source of otherwise impossible-to-find works. Thanks to the librarians there, as well as those at the Boston Public Library and the *Boston Globe*.

Finally, I want to acknowledge Hunter Flint, for being such an awesome kid, perhaps the only ten-year-old boy willing to read this book. And, to the memory of my dog Sigmund, who spent her final days by my desk. She always kept my feet—and my heart—warm during the coldest of times. You are missed.

APPENDIX

I had seen birth and death, / But had thought they were different.

—T. S. Eliot

Estimates of Number of Maternal Deaths, Lifetime Risk, Maternal Mortality Ratio, and Range of Uncertainty (2000)

	Number of maternal deaths	Lifetime risk of maternal death—1 in:	Maternal mortality ratio* (maternal deaths per 100,000 live births)
Afghanistan	20,000	6	1,900
Albania	35	610	55
Algeria	1,000	190	140
Angola	11,000	7	1,700
Argentina	590	410	82
Armenia	20	1,200	55
Australia	20	5,800	8
Austria	3	16,000	4
Azerbaijan	100	520	94
Bahamas	4	580	60
Bahrain	3	1,200	28
Bangladesh	16,000	59	380
Barbados	3	590	95
Belarus	30	1,800	35
Belgium	10	5,600	10
Belize	10	190	140
Benin	2,200	17	850
Bhutan	310	37	420
Bolivia	1,100	47	420
Bosnia and Herzegovina	10	1,900	31
Botswana	50	200	100

continued

	Number of maternal deaths	Lifetime risk of maternal death—1 in:	Maternal mortality ratio* (maternal deaths per 100,000 live births)
Brazil	8,700	140	260
Brunei Darussalam	2	830	37
Bulgaria	20	2,400	32
Burkina Faso	5,400	12	1,000
Burundi	2,800	12	1,000
Cambodia	2,100	36	450
Cameroon	4,000	23	730
Canada	20	8,700	6
Cape Verde	20	160	150
Central African Republic	1,600	15	1,100
Chad	4,200	11	1,100
Chile	90	1,100	31
China	11,000	830	56
Colombia	1,300	240	130
Comoros	130	33	480
Congo	690	26	510
Congo, Democratic Republic of the	24,000	13	990
Costa Rica	40	690	43
Côte d'Ivoire	3,900	25	690
Croatia	4	6,100	8
Cuba	45	1,600	33
Cyprus	5	890	47
Czech Republic	10	7,700	9
Denmark	3	9,800	5
Djibouti	180	19	730
Dominican Republic	300	200	150
Ecuador	400	210	130
Egypt	1,400	310	84
El Salvador	250	180	150
Equatorial Guinea	180	16	880
Eritrea	930	24	630
Estonia	5	1,100	63
Ethiopia	24,000	14	850
Fiji	15	360	75
Finland	3	8,200	6
France	120	2,700	17
French Polynesia**	—	—	—
Gabon	200	37	420
Gambia	270	31	540
Georgia	20	1,700	32
Germany	55	8,000	8
Ghana	3,500	35	540

continued

	Number of maternal deaths	Lifetime risk of maternal death—1 in:	Maternal mortality ratio* (maternal deaths per 100,000 live births)
Greece	10	7,100	9
Guadeloupe**	—	—	—
Guam**	—	—	—
Guatemala	970	74	240
Guinea	2,700	18	740
Guinea-Bissau	590	13	1,100
Guyana	30	200	170
Haiti	1,700	29	680
Honduras	220	190	110
Hungary	15	4,000	16
Iceland	—	0	0
India	136,000	48	540
Indonesia	10,000	150	230
Iran, Islamic Republic of	1,200	370	76
Iraq	2,000	65	250
Ireland	3	8,300	5
Israel	20	1,800	17
Italy	25	13,900	5
Jamaica	45	380	87
Japan	120	6,000	10
Jordan	70	450	41
Kazakhstan	560	190	210
Kenya	11,000	19	1,000
Korea, Democratic People's Republic of	260	590	67
Korea, Republic of	120	2,800	20
Kuwait	2	6,000	5
Kyrgyzstan	110	290	110
Lao People's Democratic Republic	1,300	25	650
Latvia	10	1,800	42
Lebanon	100	240	150
Lesotho	380	32	550
Liberia	1,200	16	760
Libyan Arab Jamahiriya	140	240	97
Lithuania	4	4,900	19
Luxembourg	2	1,700	28
Macedonia, Former Yugoslav Republic of	5	2,100	23
Madagascar	3,800	26	550
Malawi	9,300	7	1,800
Malaysia	220	660	41
Maldives	10	140	110

continued

	Number of maternal deaths	Lifetime risk of maternal death—1 in:	Maternal mortality ratio* (maternal deaths per 100,000 live births)
Mali	6,800	10	1,200
Malta	1	2,100	21
Martinique**	—	—	—
Mauritania	1,200	14	1,000
Mauritius	5	1,700	24
Mexico	1,900	370	83
Moldova, Republic of	20	1,500	36
Mongolia	65	300	110
Morocco	1,700	120	220
Mozambique	7,900	14	1,000
Myanmar	4,300	75	360
Namibia	190	54	300
Nepal	6,000	24	740
Netherlands	30	3,500	16
Netherlands Antilles**	—	—	—
New Caledonia**	—	—	—
New Zealand	4	6,000	7
Nicaragua	400	88	230
Niger	9,700	7	1,600
Nigeria	37,000	18	800
Norway	10	2,900	16
Occupied Palestinian Territory	130	140	100
Oman	80	170	87
Pakistan	26,000	31	500
Panama	100	210	160
Papua New Guinea	470	62	300
Paraguay	280	120	170
Peru	2,500	73	410
Philippines	4,100	120	200
Poland	50	4,600	13
Portugal	5	11,100	5
Puerto Rico	15	1,800	25
Qatar	1	3,400	7
Reunion	5	970	41
Romania	110	1,300	49
Russian Federation	830	1,000	67
Rwanda	4,200	10	1,400
Samoa**	—	—	—
Saudi Arabia	160	610	23
Senegal	2,500	22	690
Serbia and Montenegro	15	4,500	11
Sierra Leone	4,500	6	2,000

continued

	Number of maternal deaths	Lifetime risk of maternal death—1 in:	Maternal mortality ratio* (maternal deaths per 100,000 live births)
Singapore	15	1,700	30
Slovakia	2	19,800	3
Slovenia	3	4,100	17
Solomon Islands	25	120	130
Somalia	5,100	10	1,100
South Africa	2,600	120	230
Spain	15	17,400	4
Sri Lanka	300	430	92
Sudan	6,400	30	590
Suriname	10	340	110
Swaziland	120	49	370
Sweden	2	29,800	2
Switzerland	5	7,900	7
Syrian Arab Republic	780	130	160
Tajikistan	160	250	100
Tanzania, United Republic of	21,000	10	1,500
Thailand	520	900	44
Timor-Leste	140	30	660
Togo	1,000	26	570
Trinidad and Tobago	30	330	160
Tunisia	210	320	120
Turkey	1,000	480	70
Turkmenistan	40	790	31
Uganda	10,000	13	880
Ukraine	140	2,000	35
United Arab Emirates	20	500	54
United Kingdom	85	3,800	13
United States of America	660	2,500	17
Uruguay	15	1,300	27
Uzbekistan	130	1,300	24
Vanuatu**	—	—	—
Venezuela	550	300	96
Vietnam	2,000	270	130
Western Sahara**	—	—	—
Yemen	5,300	19	570
Zambia	3,300	19	750
Zimbabwe	5,000	16	1,100

*The MMRs have been rounded according to the following scheme: < 1—: no rounding; 100–999: rounded to the nearest 10; > 1,000 rounded to the nearest 100.

** No data.

Estimates developed by the World Health Organization, UNICEF, and the United Nations Population Fund.

SOURCE NOTES

My research began with some broad sources, mostly other books on the history of childbirth. Harvey Graham's *Eternal Eve,* published in London in 1950, reaches into antiquity and devotes a great deal of time to European midwifery and the outcomes of royal births. For a more modern and American perspective, there's the 1989 expanded edition of *Lying-In: A History of Childbirth in America,* by Richard and Dorothy Wertz, and Judith Walzer Leavitt's *Brought to Bed: Childbearing in America, 1750–1950,* published in 1986.

The body of work on midwifery is enormous and ranges from textbooks to polemics to biographies. For the average reader, by that I mean those looking for a book to read on the train or the beach without needing a highlighter pen, I recommend Laurel Thatcher Ulrich's *A Midwife's Tale: The Life of Martha Ballard, Based on Her Diary, 1785–1812,* and Peggy Vincent's recent autobiographical book, *Baby Catcher: Chronicles of a Modern Midwife.*

On the general topic of obstetrical history, there are two other books I would tell my girlfriends to read: *The Legacy of Dr. Lamaze: The Story of the Man Who Changed Childbirth,* written by Lamaze's granddaughter Caroline Gutmann, and *The Doctors' Plague: Germs, Childbed Fever, and the Strange Story of Ignac Semmelweis,* a gripping account written by Sherwin Nuland.

ENDNOTES

Chapter 1: Evolution and the Female Body

According to American anthropologist Wenda Trevathan: Davis-Floyd and Sargent, *Childbirth and Authoritative Knowledge*, 84.

Female members of the nomadic Pitjandjara tribe: Trevathan, 110–11.

The old woman promptly did just that: Shostak, 1–2.

According to Marjorie Shostak: Ibid., 180.

If delivery does not happen before morning: Trevathan, 78.

Humans, as well, seem to prefer: Kaiser and Halberg, 1056–68.

Also, laboring through the quiet of the night: Trevathan, 96.

Babies born late at night: Gould.

But if we had pelvises like chimps: Lewin, "Were Lucy's Feet Made for Walking?" 700.

The other shapes: Goldberg, *Ever Since I Had My Baby*, 28–29.

Polar bears: Ibid., 20.

Human babies compensate: Lewin, "The Growth of Big Brains Is Energetically Expensive," 840.

For a human baby to emerge: Montagu, 16.

"The result of these conflicting requirements": Trevathan, 22.

Doctors tried to compensate: Snow, 11.

In Australia, a 2002 report: Walker.

A headline in the Sunday Times *(London):* Harlow and O'Reilly.

Between 1920 and 1975: Wertz and Wertz, 264.

A good rule for smokers: Carrington.

Now they say: Connolly, 27–29.

Continuing on this trajectory: Trevathan, 28.

"I was gobsmacked . . .": Tozer and Hull.

Chapter 2: Midwives Throughout Time

Some oversaw sanitary conditions: Graham, 149.

European midwives: Wilson.

Some villages: Gelis, 105.

In 1600, New Amsterdam: Heaton, 607.

Sharp also recommended: Aveling, 52–53.

"No one does more harm . . .": Wiesner, 227.

Countless others were executed: Ehrenreich and English, *Witches, Midwives, and Nurses,* 7.

In 1585, two German villages: Wiesner, 220–35.

Witch hunting was so culturally ingrained: Forbes, 117.

Witch hunters believed: Wiesner, 219.

". . . not use any kind of sorcery": Graham, 176.

Three years later: Donegan, 91.

Despite Hawkins's banishment: Wertz and Wertz, 8.

The colonists deemed midwifery: Emmons, 259.

When a midwife in Guilford, Connecticut: Heaton, 607.

In 1627, Bourgeois was called: Her name was Marie de Bourbon.

Bourgeois denied the accusation: Kalish et al., 3–15.

Page—who charged six dollars per delivery: Ulrich, 177.

With midwives trained: Gelbart, 277.

At the time members of the Boston Medical Society: Litoff, 7.

Despite that initial criticism: Rooks, *Midwifery & Childbirth in America*, 19.

A physician, on the other hand: Declercq and Lacroix, "The Immigrant Midwives of Lawrence," 243.

Yet, despite being the less expensive option: DeVries, *Making Midwives Legal*, 25.

Most serious of all: Williams, 1.

"Why bother": Ibid., 6.

Not every midwife closed shop: Van Blarcom, 322–32.

"I'se got de call! . . .": Ibid., 322.

Some practiced for forty years: Logan.

So she imported nurse-midwives: Poole, 39.

Though they dealt with breeches, toxemias, and hemorrhages: Breckinridge, 314.

Breckinridge said the good results: Ibid., 315.

By 1971: "Rebirth of the Midwife," *Life,* November 1971.

Four years later: Steinman.

As baby boomers began to reproduce: Day, 72.

Two decades later: "Use of Midwives Revived in California," *New York Times,* March 20, 1973.

The California Court of Appeals: DeVries, *Making Midwives Legal,* 71.

In the Netherlands: Ibid., xvi.

But the outcomes were no worse: Declercq et al., "Home Birth in the United States," 474–82.

Chapter 3: The Hut, the Home, and the Hospital

On the Kapingamarangi atoll in Micronesia: Ashby, 185.

Ancient Egyptians: Roush, 29.

In the Auvergne region of France: Gelis, 98.

The Maori: Freedman and Ferguson, 367.

. . . and the Japanese: Carrington, 119.

The Inuits: Davis-Floyd and Sargent, *Childbirth and Authoritative Knowledge,* 448.

In sixteenth-century France: Roush, 33.

It's no wonder that Louis XIV: Bancroft-Livingston, 261–67.

"the borning room": Wertz and Wertz, 13.

The words "in the straw": Wilson, 27.

"No conversation of a depressing character": Saur, 223–28.

The staff instructed: Browne, 78.

The hospital hoped: Cody, 347.

In the position: "Rats in the Hospitals," *Harper's Weekly,* May 5, 1860, 273–74.

Logan would have been: Irving, 140–60.

He ordered that women: Wertz and Wertz, 120.

And in 1871: Browne, 249.

"The majority of patients . . .": Wertz and Wertz, 125.

When a woman giving birth: Nuland, *The Doctors' Plague,* 58.

Instead, they kept their "fatal secret": Graham, 393.

In 1843, Oliver Wendell Holmes: Nuland, *The Doctors' Plague,* 52–53.

He died in a state-run insane asylum: Cody, 312.

The surgeon-in-chief: Slemons, 93.

They later married: Nuland, *Doctors: The Biography of Medicine.*

Finally, he pressed on the abdomen: Wertz and Wertz, 137.

Equally shocking: Ibid., 161.

"The cost was such a burden . . .": Friedrich, 461.

By 1945: Tempkin, 276.

. . . in part because the federal government: Ibid., 276.

By 1954: O'Dowd and Philipp, 28.

By 1975: Davis-Floyd and Sargent, *Childbirth and Authoritative Knowledge,* 160.

The Netherlands: Kitzinger, *Birth Your Way,* 45.

"Margaret, of course, wanted breastfeeding . . .": Yans-McLaughlin, VHS.

Mead's obstetrician: Mead, *Blackberry Winter,* 249.

"And so it came about that at thirty-eight . . .": Ibid.

"According to hospital practice then": Ibid., 254-55.

"They keep her from falling off . . .": "Cruelty in the Maternity Wards," *Ladies' Home Journal,* May 1958, 45.

Although doctors have always: Warrick.

"If necessary . . .": Brody, 12.

The report concluded: Rooks et al., "Outcomes of Care in Birth Centers," 1804–11.

But still, this was mostly standard: Okun, 772.

The home births: Duran, 450–53.

There were no maternal deaths: Olson, 4–13.

A 1996 Dutch study: Wiegers, 1309–13.

Chapter 4: Pain Relief

They've been offered Demerol, Nubain, and Stadol: Carrington, 151.

The Greek goddess Actemia: Graham, 39.

And so he had this thought: Saur, 208.

The child, a boy: Wertz and Wertz, 119.

"giving her good hope . . .": Raynalde, 101.

Its intensity is almost always greater: Lieberman, *Easing Labor Pain*, 11.

"She kept saying . . .": "Cruelty in the Maternity Wards," *Ladies' Home Journal*, May 1958, 45.

Quiet has also been the norm: Jordan, 117.

Of course, most women who labor: Wertz and Wertz, 113.

"Our young women . . .": Saur, 197.

On top of that: Ibid.

A thirteenth-century Spanish alchemist: Fenster, 43.

She was so delighted: Graham, 484.

In 1591, a woman named Eufame Macalyane: Forbes, 126.

. . . and give her a potion: Lurie, 834.

King James VI: Irving, 95.

The Bible could be saying: Cohen, "After Office Hours," 896.

The biblical Paradise: Graham, 486–87.

Channing, familiar with the enduring: Caton, "Annals of Anesthetic History," 106.

The church's response: Irving, 96.

"By some divines . . .": Ibid., 97.

The woman's recovery: Channing, 159–64.

For all the drama involved: This happened on April 7, 1847.

Henry Wadsworth Longfellow's second wife: Caton, *What a Blessing She Had Chloroform*, 26.

"I never was better . . .": Kannan, 8.

"Generally, I believe . . .": Channing, 11.

In an effort to impose some standards: Leavitt, *Brought to Bed*, 123.

"If there is no one present . . .": Ibid., 121.

It was not until 1877: Caton, *What a Blessing She Had Chloroform,* 72.

By the time the woman: Graham, 488.

Her arms would be: Caton, *What a Blessing She Had Chloroform,* 135.

The doctor: Tracy and Leupp, 50.

"Give him to her": Ibid.

Women in the United States: Caton, "The Influence of Feminists."

The 'Twilight Sleep': "Mothers Discuss Twilight Sleep: Women Who Went to Freiburg for New Treatment Tell Their Experiences: Thriving Babies Exhibited," *New York Times,* November 18, 1914.

After the method migrated: Leavitt, *Brought to Bed,* 129.

One doctor said: "Doctors Disagree on Twilight Sleep," *New York Times,* August 24, 1915.

And so, on the eve of World War II: Friedrich, 461.

Cohen told the Karmels: Karmel, 38.

"You're not accustomed . . .": Ibid., 44.

She remains awake: Irving, 93.

Being unable to feel: Zhang, "Does Epidural Anesthesia Prolong Labor and Increase Risk of Cesarean Delivery?" 128–34.

Though research has shown: Wong et al.

. . . there is still great controversy: Lieberman et al., "Changes in Fetal Position."

In the UK: Nitrous oxide was discovered in England in 1824. Caton, *What a Blessing She Had Chloroform,* 92.

Chapter 5: The Cesarean Section

Not only did: Graham, 138.

If the baby's foot or arm: Young, 24–25.

Another hook: Graham, 100.

If shoulders were stuck: Ibid., 29.

Some doctors, however: Young, 51.

The scholars said: Francome, 14.

If the mother's pelvis: Young, 74.

Without the support: Speert, *Obstetric and Gynecologic Milestones*, 537.

Although Sigault had won accolades: Francome, 19.

In 1991: Ibid.

The patient reportedly recovered: Heaton, 609.

Central and South America's rates: Gomez-Dantes, 71.

She fell into a death-like sleep: Graham, 31.

His decree: Ibid., 65.

An Italian Renaissance: Ibid., 169.

The woman then had a linen pessary: Ibid.

Less than a month later: O'Dowd and Philipp, 160.

In 1785, surgeon John Aitken of Scotland: Young, 121.

The person performing the operation: Ibid., 120.

She consented: Ibid., 56.

Foster made a full recovery: O'Dowd and Philipp, 162.

Before he closed the wound: Bulletin of the History of Medicine 50 (1976): 243.

Mrs. Bennet recovered: Speert, *Obstetrics and Gynecology*, 309.

Although his patient recovered: O'Dowd and Philipp, 161.

Some doctors left the suture thread: Young, 124.

He cleaned out her insides: O'Dowd and Philipp, 163.

He then sewed the organ shut: Young, 137.

Since then: International Cesarean Awareness Network, Inc.

Before cesareans: Slemons, 87.

Although some surveys: Eide, 4–11.

Between 1970 and 1978: Cohen and Estner, *Silent Knife,* 22.

Maternal mortality: World Health Organization 2000 global maternal mortality report.

American doctors: Herrel et al., 347, 364.

These machines: Banta and Thacker, 707–19.

But in all the years of fetal monitoring: Arms, 95.

Konrad Hammacher: Ibid., 96.

They were buried together: Gorney; Remnick.

All the women: Kolder et al.

She survived: Herbert.

The hospital said: Pirani.

Out of the three million: Goldberg, *Ever Since I Had My Baby,* xv.

The weight of a pregnant uterus: Ibid., 14.

"The advocacy . . .": Leavitt, *Brought to Bed,* 64.

But a 1997 poll: Al-Mufti, 1.

An article: Sachs, 54–57.

And in 1998: Amu et al., 463.

In South Korea: Magnier.

Although a trickle of hospitals: Evans, "Caesarean: A Husband Plays Role."

"Having a father . . .": Watson.

By 1978: Smolowe.

But then, in 2002: "Committee Opinion: Induction of Labor for Vaginal Birth after Cesarean Delivery," *American College of Obstetricians and Gynecologists* 99, no. 4 (April 2002): 679–80.

Chapter 6: The Dawn of Doctors

Even by 1912: Leavitt, *Brought to Bed,* 63.

And he revived: Graham, 153.

The side position: Wertz and Wertz, 81.

He also taught: Glaister, 27.

He also bought: Ibid., 20–21.

Smellie eventually moved: Thoms, 123–24.

Even those Smellie lessons: Glaister, 56.

"As women are commonly frightened . . .": Ibid., 236.

In 1658: Graham, 257.

The other midwives: Ibid., 273–74.

If they had: Glaister, 78.

"By this admirably ingenious piece of machinery": Nihell.

"Broken barbers . . .": Ibid.

Despite Hunter's training: Leavitt, *Brought to Bed,* 102.

It is possible: Corner, 70.

Such women: Leavitt, *Brought to Bed,* 109; Corner, 70.

William Potts Dewees: In the twentieth century, feminists intellectually dissected why male birth attendants seemed more prone to the "warrior crisis response" to birth, in which a man will intervene, rescue, act, rather than use patience or gentler options more typical among midwives. Leavitt, *Brought to Bed,* 41.

. . . "Must do something": Ibid., 43.

"Conversation should be prohibited . . .": Ibid., 105.

Charles Delucena Meigs: Wertz and Wertz, 58.

"The child must not be . . .": Ibid., 112.

Sims practiced his grueling technique: Sims, 241.

We have the knowledge: LaFraniere.

DeLee's diary entry: Fishbein, 103.

American doctors: "The Operation of Episiotomy as a Prevention of Perineal Ruptures during Labor," *American Journal of Obstetrics* 11, no. 240 (1878): 517–27.

But DeLee boasted: Wertz and Wertz, 142.

"Once we can convince . . .": Fishbein, 143.

American episiotomy rates: Weber and Meyn, 1177–82; and Goldberg et al., "Has the Use of Routine Episiotomy Decreased?" 395–400.

"Look here old chap . . .": Noyes, 65.

The book, aimed at obstetricians: Dick-Read obituary, *New York Times,* June 12, 1959.

"One of the most interesting suggestions . . .": Noyes, 108.

"It was the first time . . .": Ibid., 172.

You are given the chance: Gutmann, 93.

The next morning: Ibid., 101.

"I had never seen it . . .": Lamaze, 13–14.

Pavlov's method: Wertz and Wertz, 193.

Among the forty-five hundred women: Lamaze, 188–89.

"Science and technique . . .": "Text of Address by Pope Pius on the Science and Morality of 'Painless Childbirth,'" *New York Times,* January 9, 1956.

By 1975: Flaste.

Sixty seconds after: Finster and Wood, 855–57.

Chapter 7: Tools and Fads

Physicians even bled: Leavitt, *Brought to Bed,* 44.

Although other cultures: Findley, 165.

Chamberlen, born in Paris: Carrington, 142.

He did not let: Graham, 198.

His descendants carried on: Findley, 159.

Although Mauriceau: Ibid., 315.

In 1813: Ibid., 167.

"I take pride . . .": "Complete Dilation of the Cervix Uteri, an Essential Condition to the Typical Forceps Operation," *Journal of the American Medical Association* 5 (August 29, 1885): 238–40.

"Then my hand . . .": Leavitt, *Brought to Bed,* 53.

A surgeon would insert: Wilbur, 99–104.

So Simpson took them: O'Dowd and Philipp, 149.

About fifty thousand American babies: Pope.

Babies are not born: Kitzinger, *The Complete Book of Pregnancy and Childbirth,* 230–32.

In the Yucatán: Jordan, 76.

As a bonus: Benrubi, 429–32.

And in the Auvergne region: Odent, *Entering the World,* 124.

The Siwa of Egypt: Freedman, 366–67.

Native Americans: Graham, 29.

The labor: Ibid., 148.

"Since I have adopted. . .": Thoms, 22–23.

In 1891: Benrubi, 429–32.

As many as 75 percent: Tew, 156.

"In some hospitals . . .": Chamberlain et al.

In the United States: Zhang et al., "US National Trends in Labor Induction, 1989–1998," 120–24.

Some parents and researchers: Goode.

But statistics show: Coalition for Improving Maternity Services Fact Sheet, 2003 (motherfriendly.org); Kirby, "Trends in Labor Induction in the United States," 148–51.

They gave a woman in labor: Wertz and Wertz, 137–38.

The hospital enema: Davis-Floyd, *Birth as an American Rite of Passage,* 84.

Because the study quickly: Lieberman, *Easing Labor Pain,* 187.

After doctors at Harvard: Rooks, *Midwifery & Childbirth in America,* 453.

In a 1912 letter: Leavitt, *Brought to Bed,* 60–61.

But the practice persisted: Tew, 148; Davis-Floyd, *Birth as an American Rite of Passage,* 83.

And even as late as 1993: Rooks, *Midwifery & Childbirth in America,* 454.

"Canada, French settlers . . .": Engelmann, 9.

Any disobedience: Davis-Floyd and Sargent, *Childbirth and Authoritative Knowledge,* 265, 272.

A newborn human: Odent, "What I Learned from the First Hospital Birthing Pool."

"She spent the greater part . . .": Sidenbladh, 56.

Although Charkovsky's own popularity diminished: Ibid., 59.

Odent said: Roger and Lightfoot.

In England: Laurance and Berrington.

Among all the alternative methods: Smith et al.

Greeks used slaves: Baumslag and Michels, 40.

They were also more alert: Sosa et al., 597–600.

Chapter 8: A Father's Place

In 1962 Bradley published: McCutcheon, Foreword.

His critics called him "Barnyard Bradley": Bradley.

His deception: Myles, 712.

On Lukunor: Ashby, 113.

The same was true: Ibid., 197.

After the feast: Mead, *Growing Up in New Guinea,* 72.

Even in eighteenth-century England: Cody, 343.

There were, however: Trevathan, 110.

In Ireland: Lundell.

In extreme circumstances: Gelbart, 83.

Guillemeau: Gelis, 145.

At the time: Leavitt, "Fathers in Mid-20th-Century Childbirth," 251.

In 1953: "Parents' School Ending First Year," *New York Times,* December 31, 1953.

"Sometimes it looks like": "Fathers-to-Be Don't Always Pace a Floor," *New York Times,* June 19, 1961.

Those few minutes: Goldfarb, 140–42.

In 1961: O'Dowd and Philipp, 28.

"The periodic distention . . .": Correspondence, *British Medical Journal* 594, February 25, 1961.

Why would anyone: Chandler in the final episode of *Friends.*

The decision: Wessel.

The ruling stated: Fitzgerald et al.

Some hospitals: Smolowe.

"Now we can have . . .": "Can't Bar Unwed Father, Court Says," *Toronto Globe and Mail,* May 26, 1982.

"It is never easy . . .": Taubman.

"Since the birth . . .": *Mothering,* March 1, 1996.

Being anything more: Chapman, 114–20.

"Labor coaches . . .": Herriot.

"In other cultures . . .": Trevathan, 60.

Marco Polo: Graham, 5.

Among the Arapesh: Gelis, 37.

However, with a popular culture: Hall and Dawson, *Broodmales,* 17.

A few speculated: Lundell.

Almost all of the sufferers: Brooks.

A 1985 study: Lewis.

The stress hormone: "Body & Soul," *New York Daily News,* June 30, 2004.

Many felt: Stuttaford.

"The labour . . .": "Michel Odent May Be 70 but He Is Still Making Waves," *Guardian* (London), January 18, 2000.

Chapter 9: The Postpartum Period

Louise Bourgeois: Gelis, 161–63.

Tetanus: Gordon et al., 734–42.

Delaying cord cutting: Rabe et al.

Ancient Greeks: Carrington, 135.

That practice: Thoms, 66.

The Chinese: Findley, 26.

In Transylvania: Graham, 13.

One 1980 estimate: Janszen, 78–122.

Placenta recipes: Mothering 28 (September 1983): 76.

In 1998: Beattie, "Top Chef Cooks It into Pâté," Jilly Beattie, *People,* January 18, 1998.

In 1999: "Eating Raw Human Placentas 'Risky,'" *Hong Kong Standard,* April 28, 1999.

You might think: Graham, 162.

In France: Gelis, 167.

Whether people eat: Trevathan, 106–7.

"Selling placenta is illegal . . .": Colvin and Chisholm; and Kirby.

If that was not enough of a rejuvenator: Suzuki.

In 2001: Rawe.

A key ingredient: Snead and Stratte-McClure.

Mayan mothers: Jordan, 73.

. . . and Japanese women: Findley, 28.

Some cultures believed: Davis-Floyd and Sargent, *Childbirth and Authoritative Knowledge,* 247.

In Europe: Ibid., 211.

"By the mercy of heaven . . .": Hutchinson, 102.

By 1937: Tew, 152–53.

A baby: Brozan.

"Postnatal hospital stays": Peters.

Within a month: Maryland was the first state to pass a law against drive-through deliveries. Nordheimer; McGinley, B1.

Researchers pored over: Goldberg, "Study Finds No Harm to Newborns in Short Stay."

For that rite: Wilson, 27–29.

In 1975: Flaste.

So how to facilitate: Anderson et al., "Early Skin-to-Skin Contact."

They were against wet nursing: Baumslag and Michels, 40.

In one Thai hospital: Klaus, "Mother and Infant: Early Emotional Ties," 1244–46.

And in the 1930s: Odent, Entering the World, 34.

"That tragic expression . . .": Leboyer, 6.

He would point: Ibid., 39.

"For the baby . . .": Ibid., 78.

"I don't see any logic . . .": Evans, "For Infants, Quiet and a Warm Bath."

But Leboyer baths: Anderson, "A Plea for Gentleness to the Newborn."

When someone: Ephron.

At the Dublin Foundling Hospital: Petrina Brown, 132.

In Italy: Fildes, 54.

In India: Ibid., 30.

The Catholic Church: Ibid., 105.

In the fourteenth and fifteenth centuries: Graham, 171.

Widespread news: Pfiffner, 56–59.

In New York: Klaus and Kennell, *Maternal-Infant Bonding,* 6.

"But an appeals court . . .": Angela K. Brown, "Jury Finds Yates Not Guilty."

"I was feeling so bad . . .": Shields, *Down Came the Rain,* 90.

In a rambling interview: Today, June 24, 2005. Lauer said: So postpartum depression, to you, is kind of a little psychological goo—gobbledy goop? Cruise replied: Matt, don't—no, no, I did not say that. . . . I'm not saying that isn't real. That's not what I'm saying. That's an alteration of what I'm saying. I'm saying that drugs aren't the answer. That these—these drugs are very dangerous. They're mind-altering antipsychotic drugs, and there are ways of doing it without that so that we don't end up in a brave new world. The thing that I'm saying about Brooke is that there's misinformation, okay? And she doesn't understand the history of psychiatry. She—she doesn't understand, in the same way that you don't understand it, Matt.

Shields fired back: Shields, "War of Words."

In the End

This was not a celebration: Ashby.

The book told: "Bookshelf Browsing," *American Journal of Surgery: New Series* 45 (1939): 607.

The diary of the Reverend Ezra Stiles: Wertz and Wertz, 20.

While that number: "The Midwife Throughout History," *Journal of Nurse-Midwifery* 27, no. 6 (November–December 1982): 8.

Prenatal clinics: J. W. Ballantyne, an antenatal pathology lecturer at the University of Edinburgh, is credited with preaching the value of pregnancy care, and in 1901 the Royal Maternity and Simpson Memorial Hospital began offering such services. That same year, Boston began offering home visits to pregnant women, and in 1911 the city opened its first prenatal clinic. The next year, Sydney had its first prenatal clinic. O'Dowd and Philipp, 22–23.

"Frequently the operation . . .": Hooker, 43–51.

"Little need be said . . .": DeNormandie.

In the 1930s: Slemons, 95.

By the 1960s: Drife, 311–15.

Today, according to WHO: World Health Organization, "Making Pregnancy Safer," Fact sheet no. 276, February 2004.

In France: "The Use of Incubators for Infants," *Lancet* (May 29, 1887): 1490–91.

In 1880, amid heightened concern: "The Couvreuse [sic], or Mechanical Nurse," *Lancet* 2 (August 11, 1883): 241–42.

The public: Incubated preemies were also displayed in the 1901 and 1904 World Expositions in Buffalo and St. Louis. Silverman, 127–41.

In 1912: Holt, 885–915.

Prematurity: National Center for Health Statistics.

"If mourning . . .": Klaus and Kennell, 212.

In 2003, on a morning rush-hour subway car: "Refusing Help, Woman Gives Birth aboard T," by C. Kalimah Redd and Mac Daniel, *Boston Globe,* July 31, 2003.

A more euphoric scene unfolded in 1994: Various news reports, including "Baby Born in Airplane in Critical but Stable Condition," *Orlando Sentinel,* November 29, 1994.

BIBLIOGRAPHY

Al-Mufti, R. "Survey of Obstetricians' Personal Preference and Discretionary Practice." *European Journal of Obstetrics, Gynaecology and Reproductive Biology* 73, no. 1 (1997).

Amu, O., et al. "Should Doctors Perform an Elective Caesarean Section on Request?" *British Medical Journal* 317, no. 7156 (1998): 463.

Anderson, G. C., et al. "Early Skin-to-Skin Contact for Mothers and Their Healthy Newborn Infants." *The Cochrane Database of Systematic Reviews* (2003), issue 2.

Anderson, Susan Heller. "A Plea for Gentleness to the Newborn." *New York Times*, January 15, 1978.

Anim-Somuah, M., et al. "Epidural versus Non-Epidural or No Analgesia in Labour." *The Cochrane Database of Systematic Reviews* (2005), issue 4.

Arms, Suzanne. *Immaculate Deception: A New Look at Women and Childbirth in America.* Boston: Houghton Mifflin, 1975.

Ashby, Gene, ed. *Some Things of Value: Micronesian Customs and Beliefs,* rev. ed. Eugene, OR: Rainy Day Press, 1985.

Aveling, Dr. James Hobson. *English Midwives: Their History and Their Prospects.* 1872 reprint. London: Hugh K. Elliott, 1967. A relatively short and narrowly focused book.

Bancroft-Livingston, George. "Louise de la Valliere and the Birth of the Man-Midwife." *Journal of Obstetrics and Gynaecology of the British Empire* 63 (1956): 261–67.

Banta, D. H., and S. B. Thacker. "Historical Controversy in Health Technology Assessment: The Case of Electronic Fetal Monitoring." *Obstetrics and Gynecology Survey* 56, no. 11 (November 2001): 707–19.

Baumslag, Naomi, and Dia Michels. *Milk, Money, and Madness: The Culture and Politics of Breastfeeding.* Westport, CT: Bergin & Garvey, 1995.

Benrubi, Guy. "Labor Induction: Historic Perspectives." *Clinical Obstetrics and Gynecology* 43, no. 3 (September 2000): 429–32.

Berkeley, Comyns, and Victor Bonney. *The Difficulties and Emergencies of Obstetric Practice,* 2nd ed. Philadelphia: P. Blakiston's Son, 1915.

Bernstein, Elizabeth. "Families: Divas in the Delivery Room—Moms' Demands Get Quirkier—and More Hospitals Say Yes; Placenta Art and Texas Dirt." *Wall Street Journal,* November 29, 2002.

Boisliniere, L. *Manual of Obstetric Accidents, Emergencies and Operations.* London: Henry Kimpton, 1896.

Bradley, Robert A. *Husband-Coached Childbirth,* 4th ed. New York: Bantam Books, 1996.

Breckinridge, Mary. *Wide Neighborhoods: A Story of the Frontier Nursing Service.* New York: Harper & Brothers, 1952.

Brody, Jane E. "Center for Childbirth: A Home-Like Setting." *New York Times,* September 15, 1975.

Brooks, Andrée. "Awaiting Fatherhood: The Strain." *New York Times,* December 20, 1982, sec. D.

Brown, Angela K. "Jury Finds Yates Not Guilty in Drownings." Associated Press, July 26, 2006.

Brown, Petrina. *Eve: Sex, Childbirth and Motherhood through the Ages.* Chichester, West Sussex, UK: Summersdale Publishing, 2003.

Browne, Alan, ed. *Masters, Midwives and Ladies-in-Waiting: The Rotunda Hospital 1745–1995.* Dublin: A&A Farmar, 1995.

Brozan, Nadine. "New Childbirth Center: Baby Born in Morning Was Home by Evening." *New York Times,* March 27, 1976.

Camann, William, and Kathryn J. Alexander. *Easy Labor: Every Woman's Guide to Choosing Less Pain and More Joy During Childbirth.* New York: Ballantine, 2006.

Carrington, William J. *Safe Convoy: The Expectant Mother's Handbook.* Philadelphia: J.B. Lippincott, 1944.

Caton, Donald. "Annals of Anesthetic History—Obstetric Anesthesia: The First Ten Years." *Anesthesiology* (July 1970).

Caton, Donald. "The Influence of Feminists on the Early Development of Obstetric Anesthesia." *Bulletin of Anesthesia History* (1997).

Caton, Donald. *What a Blessing She Had Chloroform: The Medical and Social Response to the Pain of Childbirth from 1800 to the Present.* New Haven, CT: Yale University Press, 1999.

Chamberlain, G., et al. *British Births 1970.* Vol. 2, *Obstetric Care.* London: Heinemann, 1978.

Channing, Walter. *A Treatise on the Etherization in Childbirth.* Boston: William D. Ticknor, 1848.

Chapman, L. L. "Expectant Fathers' Roles during Labor and Birth." *Journal of Obstetrics, Gynecology and Neonatal Nursing* 21, no. 2 (March–April 1992): 114–20.

Cody, Lisa Forman. "Living and Dying in Georgian London's Lying-In Hospitals." *Bulletin of the History of Medicine* 78 (2004): 309–48.

Cohen, Jack. "After Office Hours: Doctor James Young Simpson, Rabbi Abraham De Sola, and Genesis Chapter 3, Verse 16." *Obstetrics & Gynecology* 88, no. 5 (November 1996): 896.

Cohen, Nancy Wainer. *Open Season: A Survival Guide for Natural Childbirth and VBAC in the 1990s.* New York: Bergin & Garvey, 1991.

Cohen, Nancy Wainer, and Lois J. Estner. *Silent Knife: Cesarean Prevention and Vaginal Birth after Cesarean (VBAC).* New York: Bergin & Garvey, 1983.

Colvin, Marie, and Jack Chisholm. "Russia's Tragic Abortion Trade Fuels West's Cosmetic Industry—Roc's Wrinkle Treatments." *Sunday Times* (London), March 29, 1992.

Connolly, G., et al. "A New Predictor of Cephalopelvic Disproportion?" *Journal of Obstetrics and Gynaecology* (UK) 23 (January 2003): 27–29.

Corner, Betsey Copping. *William Shippen Jr.* Philadelphia: American Philosophical Society, 1951. A biography.

Cowhig, Jackie. "Life-Giving Water-Births." *Guardian* (UK), July 19, 1994.

Cutter, Irving S., and Henry Viets. *A Short History of Midwifery.* Philadelphia: W.B. Saunders, 1964. Oddly, this book deals only with men who were midwives.

Daniels, Karil. *Water Baby: Experiences of Water Birth.* San Francisco: Point of View Productions, 1986. VHS. A documentary film.

Datta, Sanjay. *Childbirth and Pain Relief.* Chester, NJ: Next Decade, 2001.

Davis-Floyd, Robbie. *Birth as an American Rite of Passage.* Berkeley: University of California Press, 1992. An academic book with a strong point of view.

Davis-Floyd, Robbie, and Carolyn F. Sargent, eds. *Childbirth and Authoritative Knowledge: Cross-Cultural Perspectives.* Berkeley: University of California Press, 1997.

Day, Beth. "The Return of the Midwife." *Redbook,* March 1969, 72.

Declercq, Eugene, et al. "Home Birth in the United States, 1989–1992: A Longitudinal Descriptive Report of National Birth Certificate Data." *Journal of Nurse-Midwifery* 40, no. 6 (November–December 1995): 474–82.

Declercq, Eugene, and Richard Lacroix. "The Immigrant Midwives of Lawrence: The Conflict Between Law and Culture in Early Twentieth-Century Massachusetts." *Bulletin of the History of Medicine* 159 (1985): 243.

DeLee, Joseph B. "The Prophylactic Forceps Operation." *Obstetrics and Gynecology* 1 (1920): 35.

DeNormandie, R. L. "Maternal Mortality in Boston for the Years 1933, 1934 and 1935." *New England Journal of Medicine* 216, no. 2 (January 14, 1937): 43–51.

DeVries, Raymond. *Making Midwives Legal: Childbirth, Medicine, and the Law,* 2nd ed. Columbus: Ohio State University Press, 1996.

DeVries, Raymond. *A Pleasing Birth: Midwives and Maternity Care in the Netherlands.* Philadelphia: Temple University Press, 2004.

Dick-Read, Grantly, *Childbirth without Fear.* London: Pinter & Martin, 2004.

Dick-Read, Grantly. *Natural Childbirth.* London: Heinemann, 1933.

Donegan, Jane B. *Women & Men Midwives: Medicine, Morality and Misogyny in Early America.* Westport, CT: Greenwood Press, 1978.

Drife, J. "The Start of Life: A History of Obstetrics." *Postgraduate Medical Journal* 78 (2002): 311–15.

Duran, A. M. "The Safety of Home Birth: The Farm Study." *American Journal of Public Health* 82, no. 3 (March 1992): 450–53.

Dyer, Clare. "Judge 'Wrong' in Right-to-Die Case." *Guardian* (UK), October 4, 1993.

Ehrenreich, Barbara, and Deirdre English. *Complaints and Disorders: The Sexual Politics of Sickness.* New York: Feminist Press at the City University of New York, 1973.

Ehrenreich, Barbara, and Deirdre English. *Witches, Midwives, and Nurses: A History of Women Healers.* New York: Feminist Press at the City University of New York, 1973.

Eide, M. G., et al. "Breech Delivery and Intelligence: A Population-Based Study of 8,738 Breech Infants." *Obstetrics & Gynecology* 105, no. 1 (January 2005): 4–11.

Ellison, Peter T. *On Fertile Ground: A Natural History of Human Reproduction.* Cambridge, MA: Harvard University Press, 2001.

Emmons, Arthur Brewster, II. "A Review of the Midwife Situation."
    Boston Medical and Surgical Journal 164 (1911): 259.

Engelmann, George. *Labor among Primitive Peoples*. St. Louis, MO: J.H.
    Chambers, 1882. An early anthropological classic filled with draw-
    ings of labor positions.

Ephron, Nora. "Having a Baby after 35." *New York Times*, November 26,
    1978.

Evans, Olive. "Caesarean: A Husband Plays Role." *New York Times*, Au-
    gust 18, 1976.

Evans, Olive. "For Infants, Quiet and a Warm Bath." *New York Times*,
    February 16, 1989, sec. C.

Evenden, Doreen. *The Midwives of Seventeenth-Century London*. Cam-
    bridge: Cambridge University Press, 2000. The author looked at
    twelve hundred church licensing records for midwives and, combin-
    ing those with other sources, determined that those women were not
    the poor illiterate hags history has portrayed them as.

Feinmann, Jane. "Is a Natural Birth Really Best?" *Independent* (London),
    February 23, 2004.

Fenster, Julie M. *Ether Day: The Strange Tale of America's Greatest
    Medical Discovery and the Haunted Men Who Made It*. New York:
    HarperCollins, 2001. Focuses on the first surgery with anesthesia,
    in 1846.

Fildes, Valerie. *Breasts, Bottles and Babies: A History of Infant Feeding*.
    Edinburgh University Press, 1986. Authoritative and sweeping his-
    tory of infant feeding.

Findley, Palmer. *Priests of Lucina: The Story of Obstetrics*. Boston: Little,
    Brown, 1939. A dry and not very original history.

Finster, M., and M. Wood. "The Apgar Score Has Survived the Test of
    Time." *Anesthesiology* 102, no. 4 (April 2005): 855–57.

Fishbein, Morris, with Sol DeLee. *Joseph Bolivar DeLee: Crusading Obste-
    trician*. New York: E.P. Dutton, 1949. A stunningly effusive biogra-
    phy of the Chicago obstetrician.

Fitzgerald, et al. v. Porter Memorial Hospital, U.S. Court of Appeals, 7th
    Circuit, no. 74-1949; 523 F.2d 716 (1975).

Flaste, Richard. "American Childbirth Practices." *New York Times*, No-
    vember 7, 1975.

Forbes, Thomas Rogers. *The Midwife and the Witch*. New Haven, CT: Yale

University Press, 1966. The book deals more with general superstitions than witchcraft.

Francome, Colin, Wendy Savage, Helen Churchill, and Helen Lewison. *Caesarean Birth in Britain: A Book for Health Professionals and Parents*. London: Middlesex University Press, 1993.

Freedman, Lawrence Z., and Vera Masius Ferguson. "The Question of Painless Childbirth in Primitive Cultures." *American Journal of Orthopsychiatry* 20 (1950): 363–72.

Friedrich, Lenore Pelham. "I Had a Baby." *Atlantic Monthly* 163 (1939): 461.

Gelbart, Nina Rattner. *The King's Midwife: A History and Mystery of Madame du Coudray*. Berkeley: University of California Press, 1998. The book tracks the elusive national midwife but is more broadly about the problems and struggles of midwifery in the early modern period.

Gelis, Jacques. *The History of Childbirth: Fertility, Pregnancy and Birth in Early Modern Europe*. Boston: Northeastern University Press, 1991. An English translation of a book that focuses on French birthing practices.

Ghetti, C., et al. "Physicians' Responses to Patient-Requested Cesarean Delivery." *Birth* 31, no. 4 (December 2004): 280–84.

Glaister, John. *The Life of William Smellie*. Glasgow, Scotland: Maclehose & Sons, 1894. An overly flattering biography.

Goldberg, Carey. "Study Finds No Harm to Newborns in Short Stay." *Boston Globe*, December 19, 2002.

Goldberg, J., et al. "Has the Use of Routine Episiotomy Decreased? Examination of Episiotomy Rates from 1983 to 2000." *Obstetrics and Gynecology* 99, no. 3 (March 2002): 395–400.

Goldberg, Roger. *Ever Since I Had My Baby: Understanding, Treating, and Preventing the Most Common Physical Aftereffects of Pregnancy and Childbirth*. New York: Three Rivers Press, 2003. A how-to guide for avoiding post-baby incontinence.

Goldfarb, Robert W. and Muriel. "We Shared Our Baby's Birth . . ." *Ladies' Home Journal*, December 1958, 140–42.

Gomez-Dantes, O. "Lucina's Kidnap (or How to Stop the Cesarean Section Epidemic)." *Salud Publica Mexico* 46, no. 1 (January–February 2004): 71.

Goode, Erica. "More and More Autism Cases, Yet Causes Are Much Debated." *New York Times*, January 26, 2004.

Goodwin, Karin. "Doctors and Nurses Blamed for Barriers Stopping Home Births." *Sunday Herald* (Scotland), June 1, 2003.

Gordon, John, et al. "Midwifery Practices in Rural Punjab, India." *American Journal of Obstetrics & Gynecology* (November 1, 1965): 734–42.

Gorney, Cynthia. "Whose Body Is It, Anyway? The Legal Maelstrom That Rages When the Rights of Mother and Fetus Collide." *Washington Post,* December 18, 1988.

Gould, Jeffrey B. "Evening Deliveries Have Worse Outcomes for Newborns." *Obstetrics & Gynecology* (August 2005).

Grady, Denise. "Trying to Avoid 2nd Caesarean, Many Find Choice Isn't Theirs." *New York Times,* November 29, 2004.

Graham, Harvey. *Eternal Eve.* London: William Heinemann Medical Books, 1950. A wide-ranging history focused on classical and European birth practices.

Gutmann, Caroline. *The Legacy of Dr. Lamaze: The Story of the Man Who Changed Childbirth.* New York: St. Martin's Press, 2001. Written by Lamaze's granddaughter, this book is a fascinating read that delves into the doctor's personal life.

Hall, David D. *Witch-Hunting in Seventeenth-Century New England,* 2nd ed. Boston: Northeastern University Press, 1999. An academic book mostly composed of raw witch-hunt documents.

Hall, Nor, and Warren R. Dawson. *Broodmales: A Psychological Essay on Men in Childbirth (by Hall) and the Custom of Couvade (by Dawson).* 1929. Reprint, Dallas, TX: Spring Publications, 1989. A wide-ranging anthropologic survey of couvade customs.

Harlow, John, and Judith O'Reilly. "Better British Diet Gives Birth to Mega Baby." *Sunday Times* (London), December 21, 2003.

Heaton, Claude Edwin. "Obstetrics in Colonial America." *American Journal of Surgery, New Series* 45 (1939): 606–10.

Herbert, Shiranikha. "Law Reports—Operation Authorized." *Guardian* (UK), November 3, 1992.

Herrel, Nathaly, et al. "Somali Refugee Women Speak Out about Their Needs for Care During Pregnancy and Delivery." *Journal of Midwifery and Women's Health* 49, no. 4 (July–August 2004): 345–49, 364.

Herriot, Trevor. "Birth Is Not for 'Doing.'" *Mothering,* December 22, 1994.

Holt, L. Emmett. "Infant Mortality, Ancient and Modern: An American Historical Sketch." *Archives of Pediatrics* 30 (1913): 885–915.

Hooker, Ransom S. *Maternal Mortality in New York City: A Study of All Puerperal Deaths, 1930–1932*. New York: Oxford University Press, 1933.

Hutchinson, Woods. "When the Stork Arrives." *Good Housekeeping* 59 (July 1914): 102.

Irving, Frederick. *Safe Deliverance*. Cambridge, MA: Riverside Press, 1942. A history of Boston Lying-In.

Janszen, Karen. "Meat of Life." *Science Digest* (November–December 1980): 78–122.

Jordan, Brigitte. *Birth in Four Cultures: A Crosscultural Investigation of Childbirth in Yucatan, Holland, Sweden and the United States*, 4th ed. Long Grove, IL: Waveland Press, 1993. An academic survey.

Kaiser, I. H., and F. Halberg. "Circadian Periodic Aspects of Birth." *Annals of the New York Academy of Sciences* 98 (October 30, 1962): 1056–68.

Kalish, Philip A., et al. "Louyse Bourgeois and the Emergence of Modern Midwifery." *Journal of Nurse-Midwifery* 26, no. 4 (July–August 1981): 3–15.

Kannan, Suresh. "Walter Channing and Nathan Cooley Keep: The First Obstetric Anesthetics in America." *Bulletin of Anesthesia History* (1997).

Karlsen, Carol F. *The Devil in the Shape of a Woman: Witchcraft in Colonial New England*. New York: W.W. Norton, 1998. An academic book that looks at why women were more likely to be singled out as witches.

Karmel, Marjorie. *Thank You, Dr. Lamaze*. New York: Harper & Row, 1959.

Kirby, Heather. "Something Nasty in the Night Crème? Placenta Use in Pharmaceuticals and Toiletries." *Times* (London), April 3, 1992.

Kirby, R. S. "Trends in Labor Induction in the United States: Is It True That What Goes Up Must Come Down?" *Birth* 31, no. 2 (June 2004): 148–51.

Kitzinger, Sheila. *Birth Your Way: Choosing Birth at Home or in a Birth Center*, rev. ed. London: Dorling Kindersley, 2002. Geared for general readership.

Kitzinger, Sheila. *The Complete Book of Pregnancy and Childbirth*. New York: Knopf, 2003. A general audience how-to book.

Klaus, Marshall. "Mother and Infant: Early Emotional Ties." *Pediatrics* 102, no. 5 (November 1998): 1244–46.

Klaus, Marshall H., and John H. Kennell. *Maternal-Infant Bonding: The Impact of Early Separation or Loss on Family Development.* St. Louis, MO: C.V. Mosby, 1976.

Kolder, V. E., et al. "Court-Ordered Obstetrical Interventions." *New England Journal of Medicine* 316, no. 9 (May 7, 1987): 1192–96.

Kryukova, Nine. "Born in the Waters of the Soviet Union." *Soviet Life Magazine,* June 29, 1987.

LaFraniere, Sharon. "Nightmare for African Women: Birthing Injury and Little Help." *New York Times,* September 28, 2005.

Lamaze, Fernand. *Painless Childbirth: The Lamaze Method.* Chicago: Contemporary Books, 1984. A nearly impenetrable guide to his practice.

Laurance, Jeremy, and Lucy Berrington. "Water Temperature May Have Killed Birthing Pool Baby." *Times* (London), October 16, 1993.

Leavitt, Judith Walzer. *Brought to Bed: Childbearing in America, 1750–1950.* New York: Oxford University Press, 1986. A respected, narrowly focused history.

Leavitt, Judith Walzer. "Fathers in Mid-20th-Century Childbirth." *Bulletin of the History of Medicine* 77, no. 2 (Summer 2003): 251.

Leboyer, Frederick. *Birth without Violence.* New York: Knopf, 1975. This book is practically written in poetic verse, with lots of close-cropped photos of newborns either shrieking or sleeping peacefully.

Lewin, Roger. "The Growth of Big Brains Is Energetically Expensive." *Science* 216 (May 21, 1982): 840.

Lewin, Roger. "Were Lucy's Feet Made for Walking?" *Science* 220 (May 13, 1983): 700.

Lewis, Joy Schaleben. "Symptoms of Pregnancy in Fathers-to-Be." *New York Times,* April 3, 1985, sec. C.

Lieberman, Adrienne B. *Easing Labor Pain: The Complete Guide to a More Comfortable and Rewarding Birth.* Boston: Harvard Common Press, 1992.

Lieberman, E., et al. "Changes in Fetal Position during Labor and Their Association with Epidural Analgesia." *Obstetrics & Gynecology* 105, no. 5, pt. 1 (May 2005): 974–82.

Litoff, Judy Barrett. "The Midwife throughout History." *Journal of Nurse-Midwifery* 27, no. 6 (November–December 1982): 7.

Logan, Onnie Lee, as told to Katherine Clark. *Motherwit: An Alabama Midwife's Story.* New York: E.P. Dutton, 1989. The story of Logan's life, in her own words, the book is a social history of life in the rural South, as much as a midwife's tale.

Lundell, Torborg. "Couvade in Sweden." *Scandinavian Studies* (March 22, 1999).

Lurie, S. "Ephemia Maclean, Agnes Sampson and Pain Relief during Labour in 16th Century Edinburgh." *Anesthesia* 59, no. 8 (August 2004): 834.

Magnier, Mark. "Labors of a Caesarean Culture." *Los Angeles Times*, April 19, 2001.

Marland, Hilary, ed. *The Art of Midwifery: Early Modern Midwives in Europe*. London: Routledge, 1993.

McCoy, Elin. "Birthing Rooms: Maternity Care's Newest Option." *New York Times*, May 1, 1980.

McCutcheon, Susan. *Natural Childbirth the Bradley Way*. New York: Penguin Books, 1984.

McDonald, Dearbhail. "Mega-Babies Lead to Rise in Caesareans." *Sunday Times* (London), February 6, 2005.

McGinley, Laurie. "A Family Hails Bill Providing Maternity Stay." *Wall Street Journal*, September 20, 1996, B1. Maryland was the first state to pass a law against drive-through deliveries.

McGregor, Deborah Kuhn. *From Midwives to Medicine: The Birth of American Gynecology*. New Brunswick, NJ: Rutgers University Press, 1998. An academic book that deals with J. Marion Sims.

Mead, Margaret. *Blackberry Winter: My Earlier Years*. New York: Simon and Schuster, 1972. The anthropologist's autobiography.

Mead, Margaret. *Growing Up in New Guinea*. New York: W. Morrow, 1939.

Melzack, Ronald. *The Puzzle of Pain*. New York: Basic Books, 1973. This book discusses all kinds of pain.

Montagu, Ashley. "Human Kids and Kangaroo Kids Have More in Common Than You Might Think." *Science Digest* (April 1981): 16.

Myles, Margaret F. *Textbook for Midwives*, 9th ed. Edinburgh, Scotland: Churchill Livingstone, 1981.

Nihell, Elizabeth. *A Treatise on the Art of Midwifery. Setting Forth Various Abuses therein, especially as to the practice with instruments: The whole serving to put all Rational Inquirers in a fair way of very safely forming their own judgment upon the question: In cases of pregnancy and lying-in, a man-midwife; or, a midwife*. London: A. Morley, 1760. An amazing, well-written document that seethes with contempt for male practitioners.

Nordheimer, Jon. "New Mothers Gain 2d Day in Hospital." *New York Times,* June 29, 1995, sec. B.

Noyes, Thomas A. *Doctor Courageous: The Story of Dr. Grantly Dick Read.* New York: Harper & Brothers, 1957.

Nuland, Sherwin B. *Doctors: The Biography of Medicine.* New York: Knopf, 1988.

Nuland, Sherwin B. *The Doctors' Plague: Germs, Childbed Fever, and the Strange Story of Ignac Semmelweis.* New York: W.W. Norton, 2003. A gripping story about Semmelweis's struggle to eradicate childbed fever.

Odent, Michel. *Entering the World: The De-Medicalization of Childbirth.* New York: Marion Boyars, 1984. This is translated from the original French version of *Bien Naître.*

Odent, Michel. "What I Learned from the First Hospital Birthing Pool." *Midwifery Today,* June 22, 2000.

O'Dowd, Michael J., and Elliot E. Philipp. *History of Obstetrics and Gynaecology.* New York: Parthenon, 1994.

Okun, Stacey. "Maternity with Luxury." *New York Times,* March 8, 1987.

Olson, O. "Meta-Analysis of the Safety of Home Birth." *Birth* 24, no. 1 (March 1997): 4–13.

Oxorn, Harry. *Human Labor and Birth.* New York: McGraw-Hill, Appleton & Lange, 2003.

Paget, Stephen. *Ambroise Pare and His Times: 1510–1590.* New York: G.P. Putnam's Sons, 1897.

Parvati, Jeannine. *Hygieia: A Woman's Herbal.* Joseph, UT: Freestone, 1978.

Peters, Alexandra Lally. Letter to the editor, *New York Times,* February 14, 1994.

Pfiffner, Albert. *Henri Nestle: From Pharmacist's Assistant to Founder of the World's Largest Food Company, 1814–1890.* Zurich: Chronos-Verlag, 1993. An abridged translation of the German original.

Pirani, Clara. "Mother Reported for Refusing a Caesarean." *Australian,* February 4, 2005.

Poole, Ernest. "The Nurse on Horseback Has Brought New Life and Hope to the Kentucky Mountains."*Good Housekeeping* (June 1932): 39.

Pope, Christian S. "Vacuum Extraction." *eMedicine.com,* August 17, 2004. http://www.emedcine.com/med/topic3389.htm

Rabe, H., et al. "Early versus Delayed Umbilical Cord Clamping in

Preterm Infants." *The Cochrane Database of Systematic Reviews* (2004), issue 4.

Raphael, Dana. *The Tender Gift: Breastfeeding.* New York: Schocken Books, 1976.

Rawe, Julie. "Cosmetic Placenta." *Time,* June 25, 2001.

Raynalde, Thomas. *The Byrth of Mankynde, Otherwise Named the Womans Boke.* London: T. Dawson, 1613. Translated from Latin in 1540, the earliest midwifery text printed in the English language.

Remnick, David. "Whose Life Is It, Anyway? Angie Carter Lived a Very Simple Life . . . and Died a Very Complicated Death." *Washington Post,* February 21, 1988.

Roger, Lois, and Liz Lightfoot. "Fear Grows over Water Births as More Babies Die." *Sunday Times* (London), October 17, 1993.

Rooks, Judith Pence. *Midwifery & Childbirth in America.* Philadelphia: Temple University Press, 1997. An exhaustive survey written by a respected practitioner.

Rooks, Judith Pence, et al. "Outcomes of Care in Birth Centers." *New England Journal of Medicine* 321, no. 6 (December 28, 1989): 1804–11.

Roush, Robert E. "The Development of Midwifery: Male and Female, Yesterday and Today." *Journal of Nurse-Midwifery* 24, no. 3 (May–June 1979): 29.

Sachs, B. "The Risks of Lowering the Cesarean-Delivery Rate." *New England Journal of Medicine* 340, no. 1 (1999): 54–57.

Saur, P. B. *Maternity: A Book for Every Wife and Mother.* Chicago: L.P. Miller, 1887. An early how-to guide for American women.

Sehdev, Harish. "Cesarean Delivery." *eMedicine.com,* September 22, 2004. http://www.emedicine.com/med/topic3283.htm

Shanley, Laura Kaplan. *Unassisted Childbirth.* Westport, CT: Bergin & Garvey, 1994.

Shields, Brooke. *Down Came the Rain: My Journey through Postpartum Depression.* New York: Hyperion, 2005.

Shields, Brooke. "War of Words." *New York Times,* July 1, 2005, Op-Ed.

Shostak, Marjorie. *Nisa: The Life and Words of a !Kung Woman.* New York: Random House, 1983.

Sidenbladh, Erik. *Water Babies: A Book about Igor Tjarkovsky and His Method for Delivering and Training Children in Water.* New York: St. Martin's Press, 1982.

Silverman, William A. "Incubator-Baby Side Shows." *Pediatrics* 64, no. 2 (August 1979): 127–41.

Sims, J. Marion. *The Story of My Life.* New York: Appleton and Co., 1886. The doctor's autobiography.

Slemons, J. Morris. "Progress in Obstetrics: 1890–1940." *American Journal of Surgery* 51 (1941): 79–96.

Smith, C. A., et al. "Complementary and Alternative Therapies for Pain Management in Labour." *The Cochrane Database of Systematic Reviews* (2003), issue 2.

Smolowe, Jill. "Fathers Help Out in Delivering Cesarean Babies." *New York Times,* January 8, 1978, sec. C.

Snead, Elizabeth, and Joel Stratte-McClure. "Tinseltown Spywitness." *Los Angeles Daily News,* February 27, 2005.

Snow, William. *Clinical Roentgenology of Pregnancy.* Springfield, IL: Charles C. Thomas, 1942.

Sorel, Nancy Caldwell. *Ever Since Eve: Personal Reflections on Childbirth.* New York: Oxford University Press, 1984.

Sosa, R., et al. "The Effect of a Supportive Companion on Perinatal Problems, Length of Labor, and Mother-Infant Interaction." *New England Journal of Medicine* 303, no. 11 (September 11, 1980): 597–600.

Speert, Harold. *Obstetric and Gynecologic Milestones Illustrated.* New York: Parthenon, 1996.

Speert, Harold. *Obstetrics and Gynecology: A History and Iconography.* New York: Parthenon, 2004.

Steer, Charles M. *Moloy's Evaluation of the Pelvis in Obstetrics,* 2nd ed. Philadelphia: W.B. Saunders, 1959.

Steinman, Marion. "Parent and Child: The New Old Way of Delivering Babies." *New York Times,* November 23, 1975.

Stuttaford, Thomas. "Wish You Weren't There to Begin With: Medical Briefing." *Times* (London), January 20, 2000.

Suzuki, Miwa. "Topic File: Placentas Not Wasted." *Jiji Press English News Services.* March 15, 1993.

Taubman, Philip. "Doubts in the Delivery Room." *New York Times,* October 21, 1984.

Tempkin, Elizabeth. "Rooming-In and Cold War America." *Bulletin of the History of Medicine* 76 (2002): 271–98.

Tew, Marjorie. *Safer Childbirth: A Critical History of Maternity Care.* London: Free Association Books, 1998.

Thoms, Herbert. *Classical Contributions to Obstetrics and Gynecology.* Springfield, IL: Charles C. Thomas, 1935.

Tozer, Andrew, and Liz Hull. "He's Joe-normous So Large—and Premature!" *Sunday Mail* (South Australia), March 6, 2005.

Tracy, Marguerite, and Constance Leupp. "Painless Childbirth." *McClure's Magazine* 43, no. 2 (June 1914): 37–50.

Trevathan, Wenda. *Human Birth: An Evolutionary Perspective.* New York: Aldine de Gruyter, 1987.

Trinkaus, Erik. "Neandertal Pubic Morphology and Gestation Length." *Current Anthropology* 24, no. 4 (August–October 1984): 510.

Ulrich, Laurel Thatcher. *A Midwife's Tale: The Life of Martha Ballard, Based on Her Diary, 1785–1812.* New York: Vintage Books, 1991.

Van Blarcom, Carolyn Conant. "Rat Pie: Among the Black Midwives of the South," *Harper's Monthly,* February 1930, 322–32.

Vincent, Peggy. *Baby Catcher: Chronicles of a Modern Midwife.* New York: Scribner, 2002.

Walker, Kylie. "Aust Mothers Older, Aust Babies Bigger: Report." Australian Associated Press General News, December 16, 2004.

Warrick, Pamela. "Midwives to Leave Home Denied Malpractice Insurance, Women Who Assist Home Births Face Two Choices: Go Establishment, or Go Underground." *Los Angeles Times,* April 28, 1992.

Watson, Rita E. "Making a Caesarean a Birth." *New York Times,* March 6, 1977.

Weber, A. M., and L. Meyn, "Episiotomy Rates in the United States, 1979–1997." *Obstetrics and Gynecology* 100, no. 6 (December 2002): 1177–82.

Wen, Lei H., et al. "Determinants of Caesarean Delivery among Women Hospitalized for Childbirth in a Remote Population in China." *Journal of Obstetrics and Gynaecology Canada* 25, no. 11 (November 2003): 937–43.

Wertz, Richard W., and Dorothy C. Wertz. *Lying-In: A History of Childbirth in America.* New Haven, CT: Yale University Press, 1989.

Wessel, Morris A. "Fathers Share the Nurturing Role." *New York Times,* April 1, 1990.

Wharton, Edith. *Twilight Sleep.* New York: D. Appleton and Co., 1927. A novel.

Wiegers, T. A., et al. "Outcome of Planned Home and Planned Hospital Births in Low-Risk Pregnancies: Prospective Study in Midwifery

Practice in the Netherlands." *British Medical Journal* 313, no. 7068 (November 23, 1996): 1309–13.

Wiesner, Merry E. *Women and Gender in Early Modern Europe*. Cambridge: Cambridge University Press, 1993. The book has a good chapter on witchcraft.

Wilbur, C. Keith. *Antique Medical Instruments: Price Guide Included*. West Chester, PA: Schiffer Publishing, 1987. An illustrated guide.

Williams, J. Whitridge. "Medical Education and the Midwife Problem in the United States," *Journal of the American Medical Association* 58 (January–March 1912): 1–7.

Wilson, Adrian. *The Making of Man-Midwifery*. Cambridge, MA: Harvard University Press, 1995. The author argues that male surgeons did not intend to take over births from women.

Wong, C., et al. "The Risk of Cesarean Delivery with Neuraxial Analgesia Given Early versus Late in Labor." *New England Journal of Medicine* 352, no. 7 (February 17, 2005): 655–65.

Yans-McLaughlin, Virginia. "Margaret Mead: An Observer Observed." New York: Filmmakers Library, 1995. VHS.

Young, J. H. *History of the Caesarean Section*. London: HK Lewis, 1947.

Zhang, J., et al. "Does Epidural Anesthesia Prolong Labor and Increase Risk of Cesarean Delivery? A Natural Experiment." *American Journal of Obstetrics and Gynecology* 185, no. 1 (July 2001): 128–34.

Zhang, J., et al. "US National Trends in Labor Induction, 1989–1998." *Journal of Reproductive Medicine* 47, no. 2 (February 2002): 120–24.

Organizations

American Academy of Husband Coached Childbirth (bradleybirth.com)
American College of Nurse-Midwives (acnm.org)
American College of Obstetricians and Gynecologists (acog.org)
The Coalition for Improving Maternity Services (motherfriendly.org)
DONA International (dona.org)
International Cesarean Awareness Network, Inc. (ican-online.org)
La Leche League International (lalecheleague.org)
Lamaze International (lamaze.org)
Midwives Alliance of North America (mana.org)
American Association of Birth Centers (birthcenters.org)
World Health Organization (who.int/en/)

INDEX

abortion, 247
accoucheur, 131
Acslepius, 108
Adam and Eve, 84, 85
Aegineta, Paulus, 104
Aitken, John, 111
alcohol, used for pain relief, 111, 113
alternative medicine. *See* natural medicine and folk practices
altricial infants, 17
American College of Obstetricians and Gynecologists (ACOG), 128
American Society for Psychoprophylaxis in Obstetrics (ASPO), 153, 155
analgesics, natural, 77. *See also* alcohol; morphine; opiates
Anarcha, 140
anesthesia, 84–90, 101, 152. *See also* epidural anesthesia; ether; Twilight Sleep
for cesareans, 127
harmful effects, 158–60
Virginia Apgar on, 158

animals
giving birth, 10, 11, 145, 190, 218
pelvises, 14–16
antibiotics, 226
antiseptic techniques, 42, 57, 141, 180. *See also* hand-washing
anxiety. *See* fear
Apgar, Virginia, 156, 158–60
Appalachia, 43–44
aquadural effect, 185
Arapesh, 200
Archer, Thomas, 107
Aristotle, 201
Artemis, 77
attendants. *See* birth(s), persons present at

"baby blues," 241–44
Baby-Friendly Initiative, 230
Bagryanskaya, Yekaterina, 186
Baker, Jeannine Parvati, 190–91. *See also* Parvati, Jeannine
Ballard, Martha, 37, 38
baptisms, 28, 34
Baptist Memorial Hospital, 227
barber-surgeons, 131–34, 137, 165. *See also* man-midwives